Lippincott
Photo Atlas
of Medication
Administration

Lippincott
Photo Atlas
of Medication
Administration

Sixth Edition

Pamela Lynn, EdD, MSN, RN

Assistant Professor
Gwynedd Mercy University
Frances M. Maguire School of Nursing and Health Professions
Gwynedd Valley, Pennsylvania

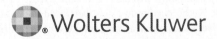

Philadelphia • Baltimore • New York • London
Buenos Aires • Hong Kong • Sydney • Tokyo

Vice President and Publisher: Julie K. Stegman
Digital Product Manager: Betsy Gentzler
Director of Product Development: Jennifer K. Forestieri
Senior Development Editor: Michael Kerns
Editorial Coordinator: Lindsay Ries
Marketing Manager: Brittany Clements
Design Coordinator: Holly Reid McLaughlin
Manufacturing Coordinator: Karin Duffield
Prepress Vendor: Aptara, Inc.

Sixth Edition

Printed in Mexico

Library of Congress Cataloging-in-Publication Data

Names: Lynn, Pamela (Pamela Barbara), 1961- author.
Title: Lippincott photo atlas of medication administration / Pamela Lynn.
Other titles: Photo atlas of medication administration
Description: Sixth edition. | Philadelphia, PA : Wolters Kluwer, [2019]
Identifiers: LCCN 2018030185 | ISBN 9781975121365
Subjects: | MESH: Drug Administration Routes | Drug Therapy–nursing |
   Pharmaceutical Preparations–administration & dosage | Atlases
Classification: LCC RM147 | NLM WB 17 | DDC 615.1022/2–dc23
LC record available at https://lccn.loc.gov/2018030185

QUADM0722

Contents

Skill 1 ▶ Administering Oral Medications

Drugs given orally are intended for absorption in the stomach and small intestine. The oral route is the most commonly used route of administration and is usually the most convenient and comfortable route for the patient. After oral administration, drug action has a slower onset and a more prolonged, but less potent, effect compared to other routes of administration.

DELEGATION CONSIDERATIONS

The administration of oral medications is not delegated to nursing assistive personnel (NAP) or to unlicensed assistive personnel (UAP) in the acute care setting. The administration of specified oral medications to stable patients in some long-term care settings may be delegated to NAP or UAP who have received appropriate training. Depending on the state's nurse practice act and the organization's policies and procedures, the administration of oral medications may be delegated to licensed practical/vocational nurses (LPN/LVNs). The decision to delegate must be based on careful analysis of the patient's needs and circumstances, as well as the qualifications of the person to whom the task is being delegated.

EQUIPMENT

- Medication in disposable cup or oral syringe
- Liquid (e.g., water, juice) with straw, if not contraindicated
- Electronic Medication Administration Record (eMAR) or Medication Administration Record (MAR)
- PPE, as indicated

ASSESSMENT

Assess the appropriateness of the drug for the patient. Review medical history, allergy, assessment, and laboratory data that may influence drug administration. Assess the patient's ability to swallow medications; check the gag reflex, if indicated. If the patient cannot swallow, is unconscious or NPO, does not have gag reflex, or is experiencing nausea or vomiting, withhold the medication, notify the primary health care provider, and complete proper documentation. Assess the patient's knowledge of the medication. If the patient has a knowledge deficit about the medication, this may be the appropriate time to begin education about the medication. If the medication may affect the patient's vital signs, assess them before administration. If the medication is for pain relief, assess the patient's pain level before and after administration. Verify the patient's name as well as the dose, route, and time of administration.

NURSING DIAGNOSIS

Determine related factors for the nursing diagnoses based on the patient's current status. Appropriate nursing diagnoses may include:

- Impaired swallowing
- Deficient knowledge
- Risk for aspiration

OUTCOME IDENTIFICATION AND PLANNING

The expected outcomes to achieve when administering an oral medication include that the medication is successfully administered via the oral route; the patient will experience the desired effect from the medication; the patient will not aspirate; the patient experiences decreased anxiety; the patient does not experience adverse effects; and the patient understands and complies with the medication regimen.

IMPLEMENTATION

ACTION	RATIONALE
1. Gather equipment. Check each medication order against the original in the medical record, according to facility policy. Clarify any inconsistencies. Check the patient's medical record for allergies.	This comparison helps to identify errors that may have occurred when orders were transcribed. The primary care provider's order or prescription is the legal record of medication orders for each facility.
2. Know the actions, special nursing considerations, safe dose ranges, purpose of administration, and potential adverse effects of the medications to be administered. Consider the appropriateness of the medication for this patient.	This knowledge aids the nurse in evaluating the therapeutic effect of the medication in relation to the patient's disorder and can also be used to educate the patient about the medication.

(continued)

Skill 1 ▶ Administering Oral Medications *(continued)*

ACTION	RATIONALE

3. Perform hand hygiene.

Hand hygiene prevents the spread of microorganisms.

4. Move the medication supply system to the outside of the patient's room or prepare for administration at the medication supply system in the medication area. Alternatively, access the medication administration supply system at or inside the patient's room.

Organization facilitates error-free administration and saves time.

5. Unlock the medication supply system or drawer. Enter pass code into the computer and scan employee identification, if required.

Locking the medication supply system or drawer safeguards each patient's medication supply. Facility accrediting organizations require medication supply systems to be locked when not in use. Entering pass code and scanning ID allows only authorized users into the computer system and identifies the user for documentation by the computer.

6. **Prepare medications for one patient at a time.**

This prevents errors in medication administration.

7. Read the eMAR/MAR and select the proper medication from the medication supply system or patient's medication drawer.

This is the *first* check of the medication label.

8. Compare the medication label with the eMAR/MAR (Figure 1). Check expiration dates and perform calculations, if necessary. Scan the bar code on the package, if required.

This is the *second* check of the label. Verify calculations with another nurse to ensure safety, if necessary.

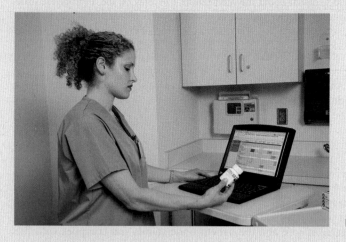

FIGURE 1. Comparing medication label with eMAR.

9. Prepare the required medications:

a. *Unit dose packages:* **Do not open the wrapper until at the bedside.** Keep opioids and medications that require special nursing assessments separate from other medication packages.

Wrapper is kept intact because the label is needed for an additional safety check. Special assessments may be required before giving certain medications. These may include assessing vital signs and checking laboratory test results.

b. *Multidose containers:* When removing tablets or capsules from a multidose bottle, pour the necessary number into the bottle cap and then place the tablets or capsules in a medication cup. Break only scored tablets, if necessary, to obtain the proper dosage. Do not touch tablets or capsules with hands.

Pouring medication into the cap allows for easy return of excess medication to the bottle. Pouring tablets or capsules into your hand is unsanitary.

ACTION

c. *Liquid medication in multidose bottle:* When pouring liquid medications out of a multidose bottle, hold the bottle so the label is against the palm. Use the appropriate measuring device when pouring liquids, and read the amount of medication at the bottom of the meniscus at eye level (Figure 2). Wipe the lip of the bottle with a paper towel.

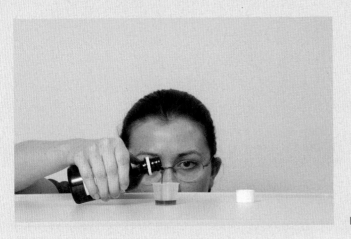

FIGURE 2. Measuring at eye level. (*Photo by B. Proud.*)

10. **Depending on facility policy, the third check of the label may occur at this point. If so, when all medications for one patient have been prepared, recheck the labels with the eMAR/MAR before taking the medications to the patient. However, many facilities require the third check to occur at the bedside, after identifying the patient.**

11. Replace any multidose containers in the patient's drawer or medication supply system. **Lock the medication supply system before leaving it.**

12. Transport medications to the patient's bedside carefully, and keep the medications in sight at all times.

13. **Ensure that the patient receives the medications at the correct time.**

14. Perform hand hygiene and put on PPE, if indicated.

15. **Identify the patient. Compare the information with the eMAR/MAR. The patient should be identified using at least two of the following methods (The Joint Commission, 2018):**

a. Check the name on the patient's identification band (Figure 3).

b. Check the identification number on the patient's identification band.

RATIONALE

Liquid that may drip onto the label makes the label difficult to read. Accuracy is possible when the appropriate measuring device is used and then read accurately.

This *third* check ensures accuracy and helps to prevent errors. *Note:* Many facilities require the third check to occur at the bedside, after identifying the patient and before administration.

Locking the medication supply system or drawer safeguards the patient's medication supply. Facility accrediting organizations require medication supply systems to be locked when not in use.

Careful handling and close observation prevent accidental or deliberate disarrangement of medications.

Check facility policy, which may allow for administration within a period of 30 minutes before or 30 minutes after the designated time.

Hand hygiene and PPE prevent the spread of microorganisms. PPE is required based on transmission precautions.

Identifying the patient ensures the right patient receives the medications and helps prevent errors. The patient's room number or physical location is not used as an identifier (The Joint Commission, 2018). Replace the identification band if it is missing or inaccurate in any way.

(*continued*)

Skill 1 ▶ Administering Oral Medications *(continued)*

ACTION	RATIONALE

ACTION

c. Check the birth date on the patient's identification band.

d. Ask the patient to state his or her name and birth date, based on facility policy.

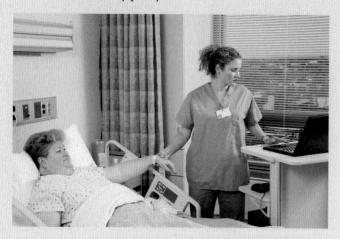

16. **Complete necessary assessments before administering medications. Check the patient's allergy bracelet or ask the patient about allergies. Explain the purpose and action of each medication to the patient.**

17. Scan the patient's bar code on the identification band, if required (Figure 4).

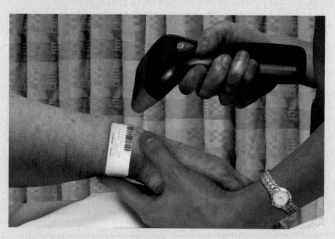

18. **Based on facility policy, the third check of the medication label may occur at this point. If so, recheck the label with the eMAR/MAR before administering the medications to the patient.**

19. Assist the patient to an upright or lateral (side-lying) position.

20. Administer medications:

   a. Offer water or other permitted fluids with pills, capsules, tablets, and some liquid medications.

   b. Ask whether the patient prefers to take the medications by hand or in a cup.

RATIONALE

This requires a response from the patient, but illness and strange surroundings often cause patients to be confused.

FIGURE 3. Comparing patient's name and identification number with eMAR.

Assessment is a prerequisite to administration of medications.

The bar code provides an additional check to ensure that the medication is given to the right patient.

FIGURE 4. Scanning bar code on patient's identification bracelet. (*Photo by B. Proud.*)

Many facilities require the *third* check to occur at the bedside, after identifying the patient and before administration. If facility policy directs the *third* check at this time, this *third* check ensures accuracy and helps prevent errors.

Swallowing is facilitated by proper positioning. An upright or side-lying position protects the patient from aspiration.

Liquids facilitate swallowing of solid drugs. Some liquid drugs are intended to adhere to the pharyngeal area, in which case liquid is not offered with the medication.

This encourages the patient's participation in taking the medications.

ACTION	RATIONALE
21. Remain with the patient until each medication is swallowed. Never leave medication at the patient's bedside (Figure 5).	Unless you have seen the patient swallow the drug, the drug cannot be recorded as administered. The patient's health record is a legal record. Medications can be left at the bedside only with a prescriber's order.

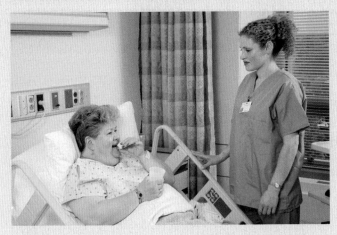

FIGURE 5. Remaining with patient until each medication is swallowed.

ACTION	RATIONALE
22. Assist the patient to a comfortable position. Remove PPE, if used. Perform hand hygiene.	Promotes patient comfort. Proper removal of PPE prevents transmission of microorganisms. Hand hygiene deters the spread of microorganisms.
23. Document the administration of the medication immediately after administration. See Documentation section below.	Timely documentation helps to ensure patient safety.
24. Evaluate the patient's response to the medication within the appropriate time frame.	The patient needs to be evaluated for therapeutic and adverse effects from the medication.

EVALUATION   The expected outcomes have been met when the patient swallows the medication, does not aspirate, verbalizes an understanding of the medication, experiences the desired effect from the medication, and does not experience adverse effects.

DOCUMENTATION

Guidelines   Record each medication immediately after it is administered on the eMAR/MAR or health record using the required format. Include the date and time of administration (Figure 6). If using a barcode system, medication administration is automatically recorded when the bar code is scanned.

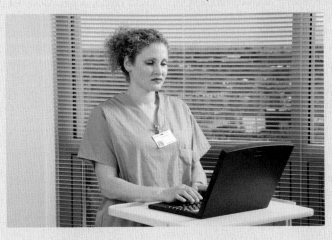

FIGURE 6. Recording each medication administered on eMAR.

(continued)

Skill 1 ▶ Administering Oral Medications *(continued)*

PRN medications require documentation of the reason for administration. Prompt recording avoids the possibility of accidentally repeating the administration of the drug. If the drug was refused or omitted, record this in the appropriate area on the medication record and notify the primary care provider. This verifies the reason medication was omitted and ensures that health care personnel providing care for the patient are aware of the occurrence. Recording administration of an opioid may require additional documentation on a controlled-substance record, stating drug count and other specific information. A record of fluid intake and output measurement is required.

Sample Documentation

DocuCare Practice documenting medication administration in *Lippincott DocuCare.*

8/6/20 0835 Patient states he is having constant stabbing leg pains. Rates pain as an 8/10. Percocet 2 tabs administered.

—K. Sanders, RN

8/6/20 0905 Patient resting comfortably. Rates leg pain as a 1/10.

—K. Sanders, RN

8/6/20 1300 Patient states he does not want pain medication, despite return of leg pain. States, "It made me feel woozy last time." Feelings discussed with patient. Patient agrees to take Percocet 1 tab at this time.

—K. Sanders, RN

8/6/20 1320 Percocet, 1 tablet given PO.

—K. Sanders, RN

UNEXPECTED SITUATIONS AND ASSOCIATED INTERVENTIONS

- *Patient states that it feels like medication is lodged in throat:* Offer patient more fluids to drink. If allowed, offer the patient bread or crackers to help move the medication to the stomach.
- *It is unclear whether the patient swallowed the medication:* Check in the patient's mouth, under tongue, and between cheek and gum. Patients with altered cognition may not be aware that the medication was not swallowed. Also, patients may "cheek" medications to avoid taking the medication or to save it for later use.
- *Patient vomits immediately or shortly after receiving oral medication:* Assess vomit, looking for pills or fragments. Do not re-administer medication without notifying the primary health care provider. If a whole pill is seen and can be identified, the primary health care provider may ask that the medication be administered again. If a pill is not seen or medications cannot be identified, do not re-administer the medication in order to prevent the patient from receiving too large a dose.
- *Child refuses to take oral medications:* Some medications may be mixed in a small amount of food, such as pudding or ice cream. Do not add the medication to liquids because the medication may alter the taste of liquids; if child then refuses to drink the rest of the liquid, you will not know how much of the medication was ingested. Use creativity when devising ways to administer medications to a child. See the section below, Infant and Child Considerations, for suggestions.
- *Capsule or tablet falls to the floor during administration:* Discard and obtain a new dose for administration. This prevents contamination and transmission of microorganisms.
- *Patient refuses medication:* Explore the reason for the patient's refusal. Review the rationale for use of the drug, explain the risk of refusal, and any other information that may be appropriate. If you are unable to administer the medication despite education and discussion, document the omission and any education and/or explanation provided related to attempts to facilitate administration according to facility policy. The primary care provider should be informed of the refusal when the omission poses a specific threat to the patient (Kee et al., 2015).

SPECIAL CONSIDERATIONS

General Considerations

- Some liquid medication preparations, such as suspensions and emulsions, require agitation to ensure even distribution of medication in the solution. Be familiar with the specific requirements for medications you are administering.

- Place medications intended for sublingual absorption under the patient's tongue. Instruct the patient to allow the medication to dissolve completely. Reinforce the importance of not swallowing the medication tablet.
- Some oral medications are provided in powdered forms. Verify the correct liquid in which to dissolve the medication for administration. This information is usually included on the package. Verify any unclear instructions with a pharmacist or medication reference. If there is more than one possible liquid in which to dissolve the medication, include the patient in the decision process; patients may find one choice more palatable than another.
- Ongoing assessment is an important part of nursing care for both evaluation of patient response to administered medications and early detection of adverse drug reactions. If an adverse effect is suspected, withhold further medication doses and notify the patient's primary care provider. Additional intervention is based on type of reaction and patient assessment.
- If the patient questions a medication order or states the medication is different from the usual dose, always recheck and clarify with the original order and/or primary care provider before giving the medication.
- If the patient's level of consciousness is altered or his or her swallowing is impaired, check with the primary care provider to clarify the route of administration or alternative forms of medication. This may also be a solution for a pediatric or a confused patient who is refusing to take a medication.
- Patients with poor vision can request large-type labels on medication containers. A magnifying lens also may be helpful.
- Provide written medication information to reinforce discussion and education in the appropriate language, if the patient is literate. If the patient is unable to read, provide written information to family or significant other, if appropriate. Written information should be at a 5th-grade level to ensure ease of understanding.
- If the patient has difficulty swallowing tablets, it may be appropriate to crush the medication to facilitate administration. However, not all medications can be crushed or altered; long-acting and slow-release drugs are examples of medications that cannot be crushed. Therefore, it is important to consult a medication reference and/or pharmacist. If the medication can be crushed, use a pill-crusher or mortar and pestle to grind the tablet into a powder. Crush each pill one at a time. Dissolve the powder with water or other recommended liquid in a liquid medication cup, keeping each medication separate from the others. Keep the package label with the medication cup for future comparison of information. Combine the crushed medication with a small amount of soft food, such as applesauce or pudding, to facilitate administration.

Infant and Child Considerations

- Special devices, such as oral syringes and calibrated nipples, are available in a pharmacy to ensure accurate dose calculations for young children and infants.
- Some creative ways to administer medications to children include the following: have a "tea party" with medicine cups; place oral syringe (without needle) or dropper in the space between the cheek and gum and slowly administer the medication; save a special treat for after the medication administration (e.g., movie, playroom time, or a special food, if allowed).
- If a medication has an objectionable taste, warn the child if he or she is old enough to understand. Failing to warn the child is likely to decrease the child's trust in the nurse. Do not lie to a child about medication administration.
- Caution caregivers to remove and dispose of plastic syringe caps present on the end of syringes before drug administration to reduce the risk of choking. Companies manufacture syringes labeled "oral use" without the caps on them and should be considered for use (Grissinger, 2014; ISMP, 2012b).

Older Adult Considerations

- Older adults with arthritis may have difficulty opening childproof caps. On request, the pharmacist can substitute a cap that is easier to open. A rubber band twisted around the cap may provide a more secure grip for older adults.
- Consider large-print written medication information, when appropriate.
- Physiologic changes associated with the aging process, including decreased gastric motility, muscle mass, acid production, and blood flow, can affect patient's response to medication, including drug absorption and increased risk of adverse effects. Older adults are more likely to take multiple drugs, so drug interactions in the older adult are a very real and dangerous problem (Adams et al., 2017).

(continued)

Skill 1 ▶ Administering Oral Medications *(continued)*

Home Care Considerations

- Encourage the patient to discard expired prescription medications based on label instructions or community guidelines.
- Discuss safe storage of medications when there are children and pets in the home environment.
- Discuss with parents the difference in over-the-counter medications made for infants and medications made for children. Many times parents do not realize that there are different strengths to the actual medications, leading to under- or overdosing.
- Encourage patients to carry a card listing all medications they take, including dosage and frequency, in case of an emergency.
- Discuss the importance of using an appropriate measuring device for liquid medications. Caution patients not to use eating utensils for measuring medications; use a liquid medication cup, oral syringe, or measuring spoon to provide accurate dosing.

EVIDENCE FOR PRACTICE ▶

MEDICATION ERRORS

Medication errors occur frequently and are a serious problem in health care. Medication errors may have serious consequences. Health care providers, including nurses, have a responsibility to prevent medication errors. What nursing practices may help improve the medication administration process?

Related Research

Niemann, D., Bertsche, A., Meyrath, D., et al. (2015). A prospective three-step intervention study to prevent medication errors in drug handling in paediatric care. *Journal of Clinical Nursing, 24*(1/2), 101–114.

This study investigated errors in drug handling by pediatric nurses on one unit of a university children's hospital. Medication errors on the unit were tracked before the intervention to provide a baseline. Errors were tracked again after the three steps of the intervention were completed. Four pharmacists, trained to monitor and document drug-handling processes using a developed checklist, monitored drug handling during morning medication administration for 20 working days. Each error on the checklist was assessed in an independent survey by an expert panel and assigned a clinical relevance value. Following baseline monitoring, nurse participants completed a survey to detect their knowledge regarding drug handling. Each nurse then participated in three education interventions, with content based on individual responses to the questionnaire. Nursing education targeting different causes of errors included a three-page handout addressing knowledge deficits; an hour-long training course addressing errors caused by rule violations and slips; and a comprehensive reference book addressing knowledge-, memory-, and rule-based errors. A total of 37 nurses, including 14 student nurses, agreed to participate, and 83% of the licensed participants specialized in pediatric care. Medications were administered to a total of 195 patients during the four monitoring periods, with a total of 1,920 drug-handling processes. The number of patients subjected to at least one medication error in drug handling decreased from 88% at baseline to 49% after the third intervention. The overall frequency of errors decreased form 91% to 26%. The authors concluded that interventions targeting the different causes of errors is an effective means to reduce medication errors and must be multifactorial.

Relevance to Nursing Practice

Medication administration is an important nursing responsibility. Nurses need to be aware of the factors that contribute to medication errors and work to reduce these factors in their practice. Nurses have a responsibility to be familiar with, and conform to, facility policies, as well as to maintain professional competency in regard to current and best practice guidelines.

Skill 2 ▶ Administering Medications via a Gastric Tube

Patients with a gastrointestinal tube (nasogastric, nasointestinal, percutaneous endoscopic gastrostomy [PEG], or jejunostomy [J] tube) often receive medication through the tube. Care of the patient with an enteral feeding tube. Use liquid medications, when possible, because they are readily absorbed and less likely to cause tube occlusions. Dilute thick suspensions as recommended (Bankhead et al., 2009; Best & Wilson, 2011). Certain solid dosage medications can be crushed and combined with liquid. Crush each pill, one at a time, grinding to a fine powder and mix with 15 to 30 mL of water before delivery through the tube, keeping each medication separate from the others and flushing with water between each medication. The medications may not be physically or chemically compatible; mixing them can lead to tube obstruction or altered therapeutic actions (Bankhead et al.; Best & Wilson). Some sources recommend sterile water for medication administration, as the chemical contaminants in tap water can potentiate drug–drug interactions (Bankhead et al.). In addition, sterile water should be used for tube flushes in immunocompromised or critically ill patients (Bankhead et al.; Allen, 2015).

Certain capsules may be opened, emptied into liquid, and administered through the tube (Williams, 2008). **Not all medications can be crushed or altered; long-acting and slow-release drugs are examples of medications that cannot be crushed.** Check manufacturer's recommendations and/or with a pharmacist to verify. In addition, the absorption (e.g., phenytoin) and/or effect (carbidopa/levodopa) of some medications are altered when co-administered with enteral feeding formulas (Zhu & Zhou, 2013). Nurses must know procedures for and the latest evidence on drug administration by nasogastric and gastric tubes (Zhu & Zhou). Once prepared, keep the package label with the medication cup for future comparison of information.

DELEGATION CONSIDERATIONS

The administration of medications via a gastric tube is not delegated to nursing assistive personnel (NAP) or to unlicensed assistive personnel (UAP). Depending on the state's nurse practice act and the organization's policies and procedures, the administration of medications via a gastric tube may be delegated to licensed practical/vocational nurses (LPN/LVNs). The decision to delegate must be based on careful analysis of the patient's needs and circumstances, as well as the qualifications of the person to whom the task is being delegated.

EQUIPMENT

- Irrigation set (60-mL syringe and irrigation container)
- Medications
- Tap water or sterile water (or normal saline), for irrigation, depending on facility policy
- Gloves
- Additional PPE, as indicated

ASSESSMENT

Assess the appropriateness of the drug for the patient. Review medical history, allergy, assessment, and laboratory data that may influence drug administration. Research each medication to be given, especially for mode of action, side effects, nursing implications, ability to be crushed, and whether the medication should be given with or without food. Verify patient name, dose, route, and time of administration. Assess patient's knowledge of the medication and the reason for its administration. If the patient has a knowledge deficit about the medication, this may be the appropriate time to begin educating the patient about the medication. Auscultate the abdomen for evidence of bowel sounds. Palpate the abdomen for tenderness and distention. Ascertain the time of the patient's last bowel movement and measure abdominal girth, if appropriate. If the medication may affect the patient's vital signs, assess them before administration. If the medication is for pain relief, assess the patient's pain level before and after administration.

(continued)

Skill 2 ▶ Administering Medications via a Gastric Tube *(continued)*

NURSING DIAGNOSIS	Determine the related factors for the nursing diagnoses based on the patient's current status. Possible nursing diagnoses may include: • Deficient knowledge • Risk for aspiration • Risk for injury
OUTCOME IDENTIFICATION AND PLANNING	The expected outcome to achieve is that the patient receives the medication via the tube and experiences the intended effect of the medication. In addition, the patient verbalizes knowledge of the medications given; the patient remains free from adverse effects and injury; and the gastric tube remains patent.

IMPLEMENTATION

ACTION	RATIONALE
1. Gather equipment. Check each medication order against the original in the medical record, according to facility policy. Clarify any inconsistencies. Check the patient's health record for allergies.	This comparison helps to identify errors that may have occurred when orders were transcribed. The primary care provider's order or prescription is the legal record of medication orders for each facility.
2. Know the actions, special nursing considerations, safe dose ranges, purpose of administration, and adverse effects of the medications to be administered. Consider the appropriateness of the medication for this patient.	This knowledge aids the nurse in evaluating the therapeutic effect of the medication in relation to the patient's disorder and can also be used to educate the patient about the medication.
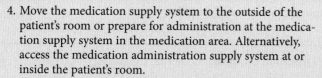 3. Perform hand hygiene.	Hand hygiene prevents the spread of microorganisms.
4. Move the medication supply system to the outside of the patient's room or prepare for administration at the medication supply system in the medication area. Alternatively, access the medication administration supply system at or inside the patient's room.	Organization facilitates error-free administration and saves time.
5. Unlock the medication supply system or drawer. Enter pass code into the computer and scan employee identification, if required.	Locking the medication supply system or drawer safeguards each patient's medication supply. Facility accrediting organizations require medication supply systems to be locked when not in use. Entering pass code and scanning ID allows only authorized users into the computer system and identifies the user for documentation by the computer.
6. **Prepare medications for one patient at a time.**	This prevents errors in medication administration.
7. Read the eMAR/MAR and select the proper medication from the medication supply system or patient's medication drawer.	This is the *first* check of the label.
8. Compare the label with the eMAR/MAR. Check expiration dates and perform calculations, if necessary. Scan the bar code on the package, if required.	This is the *second* check of the label. Verify calculations with another nurse to ensure safety, if necessary.
9. Check to see if medications to be administered come in a liquid form. **If pills or capsules are to be given, check with pharmacy or drug reference to verify the ability to crush tablets or open capsules.**	To prevent the tube from becoming clogged, all medications should be given in liquid form whenever possible. Medications in extended-release formulations should not be crushed before administration.

ACTION	**RATIONALE**

10. Prepare medication.

   Pills: Using a pill crusher, crush each pill one at a time. Dissolve the powder with water or other recommended liquid in a liquid medication cup, keeping each medication separate from the others. Keep the package label with the medication cup, for future comparison of information.

Some medications require dissolution in liquid other than water. The medications may not be physically or chemically compatible; mixing them can lead to tube obstruction or altered therapeutic actions (Bankhead et al., 2009; Best & Wilson, 2011). The label is needed for an additional safety check. Some medications require pre-administration assessments.

   Liquid: When pouring liquid medications from a multidose bottle, hold the bottle with the label against the palm. Use the appropriate measuring device when pouring liquids, and read the amount of medication at the bottom of the meniscus at eye level (Refer to Step 9c in Skill 1). Wipe the lip of the bottle with a paper towel.

Liquid that may drip onto the label makes the label difficult to read. Accuracy is possible when the appropriate measuring device is used and then read accurately.

11. **Depending on facility policy, the third check of the label may occur at this point. If so, when all medications for one patient have been prepared, recheck the labels with the eMAR/MAR before taking the medications to the patient. However, many facilities require the third check to occur at the bedside, after identifying the patient.**

This *third* check ensures accuracy and helps to prevent errors. *Note:* Many facilities require the *third* check to occur at the bedside, after identifying the patient and before administration.

12. Replace any multidose containers in the patient's drawer or medication supply system.

Proper storage safeguards medications.

13. **Lock the medication supply system before leaving it.**

Locking the medication supply system or drawer safeguards the patient's medication supply. Facility accrediting organizations require medication supply systems to be locked when not in use.

14. Transport medications to the patient's bedside carefully, and keep the medications in sight at all times.

Careful handling and close observation prevent accidental or deliberate disarrangement of medications.

15. **Ensure that the patient receives the medications at the correct time.**

Check facility policy, which may allow for administration within a period of 30 minutes before or 30 minutes after the designated time.

16. Perform hand hygiene and put on PPE, if indicated.

Hand hygiene and PPE prevent the spread of microorganisms. PPE is required based on transmission precautions.

17. **Identify the patient. Compare the information with the eMAR/MAR. The patient should be identified using at least two of the following methods (The Joint Commission, 2018):**

Identifying the patient ensures the right patient receives the medications and helps prevent errors. The patient's room number or physical location is not used as an identifier (The Joint Commission, 2018). Replace the identification band if it is missing or inaccurate in any way.

   a. Check the name on the patient's identification band.

   b. Check the identification number on the patient's identification band.

This requires a response from the patient, but illness and strange surroundings often cause patients to be confused.

   c. Check the birth date on the patient's identification band.

   d. Ask the patient to state his or her name and birth date, based on facility policy.

18. **Complete necessary assessments before administering medications. Check the patient's allergy bracelet or ask the patient about allergies. Explain what you are going to do, and the reason for doing it, to the patient.**

Assessment is a prerequisite to administration of medications. Explanation relieves anxiety and facilitates cooperation.

(continued)

Skill 2 ▶ Administering Medications via a Gastric Tube *(continued)*

ACTION	RATIONALE
19. Scan the patient's bar code on the identification band, if required (Figure 1).	This provides an additional check to ensure that the medication is given to the right patient.
20. **Based on facility policy, the third check of the label may occur at this point. If so, recheck the labels with the eMAR/MAR before administering the medications to the patient.**	Many facilities require the *third* check to occur at the bedside, after identifying the patient and before administration. If facility policy directs the *third* check at this time, this *third* check ensures accuracy and helps to prevent errors.
21. Assist the patient to the high-Fowler's position, unless contraindicated.	This reduces the risk of aspiration.
22. Put on gloves.	Gloves prevent contact with mucous membranes and body fluids.
23. If patient is receiving continuous tube feedings, pause the tube-feeding pump (Figure 2).	If the pump is not stopped, tube feeding will flow out of the tube and onto the patient.

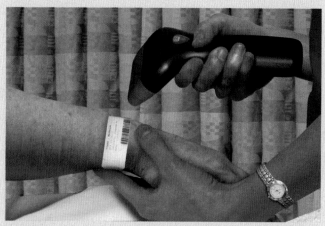

FIGURE 1. Scanning bar code on the patient's identification bracelet. (*Photo by B. Proud.*)

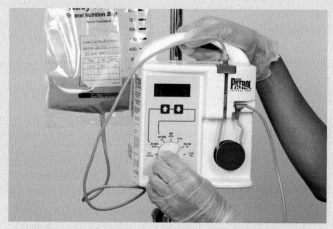

FIGURE 2. Pausing feeding pump. (*Photo by B. Proud.*)

24. Pour the water into the irrigation container. Measure 30 mL of water. Apply clamp on feeding tube, if present. Alternatively, pinch gastric tube below port with fingers, or position stopcock to correct direction. Open port on gastric tube delegated to medication administration (Figure 3) or disconnect tubing for feeding from gastric tube and place cap on end of feeding tubing.	Fluid is ready for flushing of the tube. Applying clamp, folding the tube over, and clamping, or the correct positioning of the stopcock prevents any backflow of gastric drainage. Covering end of feeding tubing prevents contamination.

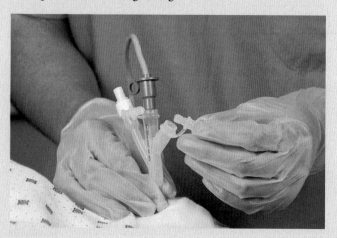

FIGURE 3. Pinching gastric tubing to prevent backflow of gastric drainage and opening medication administration port. (*Photo by B. Proud.*)

ACTION

RATIONALE

25. **Check tube placement, depending on type of tube and facility policy.**

Tube placement must be confirmed before administering anything through the tube to avoid inadvertent instillation in the respiratory tract.

26. Note the amount of any residual. Replace residual back into stomach, based on facility policy.

Research findings are inconclusive on the benefit of returning gastric volumes to the stomach or intestine to avoid fluid or electrolyte imbalance, which has been accepted practice. Consult facility policy concerning this practice.

27. Apply clamp on feeding tube, if present. Alternatively, pinch the gastric tube below port with fingers, or position stop-cock to correct direction. Remove 60-mL syringe from gastric tube. Remove the plunger of the syringe. Reinsert the syringe in the gastric tube without the plunger. Pour 30 mL of water into the syringe (Figure 4). **Unclamp the tube and allow the water to enter the stomach via gravity infusion.**

Clamping prevents backflow of gastric drainage. Flushing the tube ensures that all the residual is cleared from the tube.

28. Administer the first dose of medication by pouring it into the syringe (Figure 5). Follow with a 5- to 10-mL water flush between medication doses. Follow the last dose of medication with 30 to 60 mL of water flush.

Flushing between medications prevents any possible interactions between the medications. Flushing at the end maintains tube patency, prevents blockage by medication particles, and ensures all doses enter the stomach.

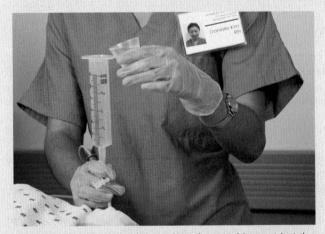

FIGURE 4. Pouring water into syringe inserted in gastric tube. (*Photo by B. Proud.*)

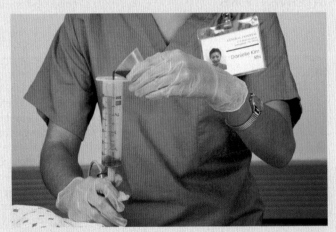

FIGURE 5. Pouring medication into syringe inserted in gastric tube. (*Photo by B. Proud.*)

29. Clamp the tube, remove the syringe, and replace the feeding tubing. If a stopcock is used, position it to correct direction. If a tube medication port was used, cap the port. Unclamp the gastric tube and restart tube feeding, if appropriate for medications administered.

Some medications require the holding of the tube feeding for a certain period of time after administration. Consult a drug reference or a pharmacist.

30. Remove gloves. Assist the patient to a comfortable position. If receiving a tube feeding, the head of the bed must remain elevated at least 30 degrees.

Ensures patient comfort. Keeping the head of the bed elevated helps prevent aspiration.

31. Remove additional PPE, if used. Perform hand hygiene.

Proper removal of PPE reduces the risk for infection transmission and contamination of other items. Hand hygiene prevents the spread of microorganisms.

32. Document the administration of the medication immediately after administration. See Documentation section below.

Timely documentation helps to ensure patient safety.

33. Evaluate the patient's response to the medication within the appropriate time frame.

The patient needs to be evaluated for therapeutic and adverse effects from the medication.

(*continued*)

Skill 2 ▸ Administering Medications via a Gastric Tube *(continued)*

EVALUATION

The expected outcome has been met when the patient receives the prescribed medications and experiences the intended effects of the medications administered. In addition, the patient demonstrates a patent and functioning gastric tube, verbalizes knowledge of the medications given, and remains free from adverse effects and injury.

DOCUMENTATION

Guidelines

Document the administration of the medication immediately after administration, including date, time, dose, and route of administration on the eMAR/MAR or record using the required format. If using a bar-code system, medication administration is automatically recorded when the bar code is scanned. PRN medications require documentation of the reason for administration. Prompt recording avoids the possibility of accidentally repeating the administration of the drug. Record the amount of gastric residual, if appropriate. Record the amount of liquid given on the intake and output record. If the drug was refused or omitted, record this in the appropriate area on the medication record and notify the primary care provider. This verifies the reason medication was omitted and ensures that health care personnel providing care for the patient are aware of the occurrence.

UNEXPECTED SITUATIONS AND ASSOCIATED INTERVENTIONS

- *Medication enters tube and then tube becomes clogged:* Attach a 60-mL syringe onto end of tube. Pull back and then lightly apply pressure to plunger in a repetitive motion. This may dislodge the medication. Try using warm water or air and gentle pressure to remove the clog. Carbonated sodas, such as colas, and meat tenderizers have not been shown effective in removing clogs in feeding tubes. Never use a stylet to unclog tubes. If the medication does not move through the tube, notify the primary care provider. The tube may have to be replaced.

SPECIAL CONSIDERATIONS

- If medications are being administered via an NG tube that is attached to suction, the tube should remain clamped, off suction, for a period of time after medication administration. This allows for medication absorption before returning to suction. Check facility policy and drug reference for specific drug requirements.
- If necessary to use plunger in irrigation syringe to administer medications, instill gently and slowly. Gravity administration is considered best to avoid excess pressure.
- Give medications separately and flush with water between each drug. Some medications may interact with each other or become less effective if mixed with other drugs.
- If the patient is receiving tube feedings, review information about the drugs to be administered. Absorption of some drugs, such as phenytoin, is affected by tube feeding formulas. Discontinue a continuous tube feeding and leave the tube clamped for the required period of time before and after the medication has been given, according to the reference and facility protocol.
- Ongoing assessment is an important part of nursing care for both evaluation of patient response to administered medications and early detection of adverse drug reactions. If an adverse effect is suspected, withhold further medication doses and notify the patient's primary care provider. Additional intervention is based on type of reaction and patient assessment.

Skill 3 ▸ Removing Medication From an Ampule

An **ampule** is a glass flask that contains a single dose of medication for parenteral administration. Because there is no way to prevent contamination of any unused portion of medication after the ampule is opened, discard any remaining medication if not all the medication is used for the prescribed dose. You must break the thin neck of the ampule to remove the medication.

DELEGATION CONSIDERATIONS

The preparation of medication from an ampule is not delegated to nursing assistive personnel (NAP) or to unlicensed assistive personnel (UAP). Depending on the state's nurse practice act and the organization's policies and procedures, the preparation of medication from an ampule may be delegated to a licensed practical/vocational nurse (LPN/LVN). The decision to delegate must be based on careful analysis of the patient's needs and circumstances, as well as the qualifications of the person to whom the task is being delegated.

EQUIPMENT	• Sterile syringe and filter needle • Ampule of medication • Antimicrobial swab • Small, sterile gauze pad • Electronic Medication Administration Record (eMAR) or Medication Administration Record (MAR)

ASSESSMENT

Assess the appropriateness of the drug for the patient. Review medical history, allergy, assessment, and laboratory data that may influence drug administration. Assess the medication in the ampule for any particles or discoloration. Assess the ampule for any cracks or chips. Check expiration date before administering the medication. Verify patient name, dose, route, and time of administration.

NURSING DIAGNOSIS

Determine related factors for the nursing diagnoses based on the patient's current status. Appropriate nursing diagnoses may include:

• Risk for infection
• Deficient knowledge
• Risk for injury

OUTCOME IDENTIFICATION AND PLANNING

The expected outcome to achieve when removing medication from an ampule is that the medication is removed in a sterile manner; the medication is free from glass shards and contamination; and the proper dose prepared.

IMPLEMENTATION

ACTION	**RATIONALE**
1. Gather equipment. Check the medication order against the original order in the medical record, according to facility policy. Clarify any inconsistencies. Check the patient's health record for allergies.	This comparison helps to identify errors that may have occurred when orders were transcribed. The primary care provider's order or prescription is the legal record of medication orders for each facility.
2. Know the actions, special nursing considerations, safe dose ranges, purpose of administration, and adverse effects of the medications to be administered. Consider the appropriateness of the medication for this patient.	This knowledge aids the nurse in evaluating the therapeutic effect of the medication in relation to the patient's disorder and can also be used to educate the patient about the medication.
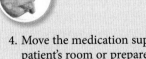3. Perform hand hygiene.	Hand hygiene prevents the spread of microorganisms.
4. Move the medication supply system to the outside of the patient's room or prepare for administration at the medication supply system in the medication area. Alternatively, access the medication administration supply system at or inside the patient's room.	Organization facilitates error-free administration and saves time.
5. Unlock the medication supply system or drawer. Enter pass code and scan employee identification, if required.	Locking the medication supply system or drawer safeguards each patient's medication supply. Facility accrediting organizations require medication supply systems to be locked when not in use. Entering pass code and scanning ID allows only authorized users into the computer system and identifies the user for documentation by the computer.

(continued)

Skill 3 ▶ Removing Medication From an Ampule *(continued)*

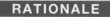

ACTION	RATIONALE
6. **Prepare medications for one patient at a time.**	This prevents errors in medication administration.
7. Read the eMAR/MAR and select the proper medication from the medication supply system or the patient's medication drawer.	This is the *first* check of the label.
8. Compare the label with the eMAR/MAR. Check expiration dates and perform calculations, if necessary. Scan the bar code on the package, if required.	This is the *second* check of the label. Verify calculations with another nurse to ensure safety, if necessary.
9. Tap the stem of the ampule (Figure 1) or twist your wrist quickly (Figure 2) while holding the ampule vertically.	This facilitates movement of medication in the stem to the body of the ampule.

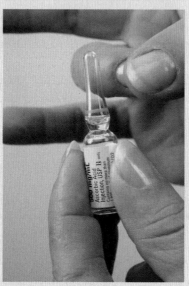

FIGURE 1. Tapping stem of the ampule.

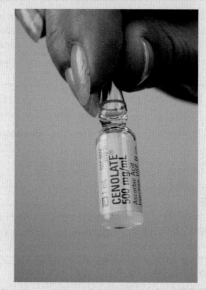

FIGURE 2. Twisting wrist quickly while holding ampule vertically.

10. Using the antimicrobial swab, scrub the neck of the ampule (Dolan et al, 2016). Wrap a small sterile gauze pad around the neck of the ampule.	Scrubbing the neck is necessary to reduce the risk of contamination (Dolan et al., 2016). Wrapping the neck of the ampule with gauze protects your fingers from the glass as the ampule is broken.
11. Breaking away from your body, use a snapping motion to break off the top of the ampule along the scored line at its neck (Figure 3). **Always break away from your body.**	This protects your face and fingers from any shattered glass fragments.

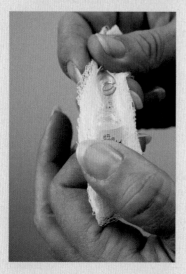

FIGURE 3. Using a snapping motion to break top of ampule.

ACTION

12. Attach filter needle to syringe. Remove the cap from the filter needle by pulling it straight off.

13. Withdraw medication in the amount ordered plus a small amount more (approximately 30% more). **Do not inject air into the solution. While inserting the filter needle into the ampule, be careful not to touch the rim.** Use either of the following methods to withdraw the medication:

    a. Insert the tip of the needle into the ampule, which is upright on a flat surface, and withdraw fluid into the syringe (Figure 4). **Touch the plunger only at the knob.**

    b. Insert the tip of the needle into the ampule and invert the ampule. Keep the needle centered and not touching the sides of the ampule. Withdraw fluid into syringe (Figure 5). **Touch the plunger only at the knob.**

RATIONALE

Use of a filter needle prevents the accidental withdrawing of small glass particles with the medication. Pulling the cap off in a straight manner prevents accidental needlestick.

By withdrawing an additional small amount of medication, any air bubbles in the syringe can be displaced once the syringe is removed while allowing ample medication to remain in the syringe. The contents of the ampule are not under pressure; therefore, air is unnecessary and will cause the contents to overflow. The rim of the ampule is considered contaminated.

Handling the plunger only at the knob will keep the shaft of the plunger sterile.

Surface tension holds the fluids in the ampule when inverted. If the needle touches the sides or is removed and then reinserted into the ampule, surface tension is broken, and fluid runs out. Handling the plunger only at the knob will keep the shaft of the plunger sterile.

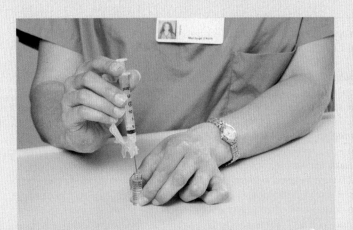

FIGURE 4. Withdrawing medication from upright ampule. (*Photo by B. Proud.*)

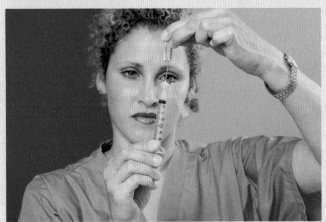

FIGURE 5. Withdrawing medication from inverted ampule. (*Photo by B. Proud.*)

14. Wait until the needle has been withdrawn to tap the syringe and expel the air carefully by pushing on the plunger. **Check the amount of medication in the syringe with the medication dose and discard any surplus, according to facility policy.**

15. **Depending on facility policy, the third check of the label may occur at this point. If so, when all medications for one patient have been prepared, recheck the labels with the eMAR/MAR before taking the medications to the patient. However, many facilities require the third check to occur at the bedside, after identifying the patient.**

16. **Engage safety guard on filter needle and remove the needle. Discard the filter needle in a suitable container. Attach appropriate administration device to syringe.**

17. Discard the ampule in a suitable container.

Ejecting air into the solution increases pressure in the ampule and can force the medication to spill out over the ampule. Ampules may have overfill. Careful measurement ensures that the correct dose is withdrawn.

This *third* check ensures accuracy and helps to prevent errors. *Note:* Many facilities require the *third* check to occur at the bedside, after identifying the patient and before administration.

The filter needle used to draw up medication should not be used to administer the medication. This will prevent any glass shards from entering the patient during administration.

Any medication that has not been removed from the ampule must be discarded because sterility of contents cannot be maintained in an opened ampule.

(continued)

Skill 3 ▶ Removing Medication From an Ampule *(continued)*

ACTION	RATIONALE
18. Lock the medication supply system before leaving it.	Locking the medication supply system safeguards the patient's medication supply. Facility accrediting organizations require medication supply systems to be locked when not in use.
19. Perform hand hygiene.	Hand hygiene deters the spread of microorganisms.
20. Proceed with administration, based on prescribed route.	See appropriate skill for prescribed route.

EVALUATION

The expected outcomes have been met when the medication is removed from the ampule in a sterile manner, is free from glass shards, and the proper dose is prepared.

DOCUMENTATION

Guidelines

It is not necessary to record the removal of the medication from the ampule. Prompt recording of administration of the medication is required immediately after it is administered.

UNEXPECTED SITUATIONS AND ASSOCIATED INTERVENTIONS

- *You cut yourself while trying to open the ampule:* Discard ampule and medication in case contamination has occurred. Clean and bandage the wound and obtain a new ampule. Report incident according to facility policy.
- *All of medication was not removed from the stem and insufficient medication remains in body of ampule for dose:* Discard ampule and drawn medication. Obtain a new ampule and start over. Medication in original ampule stem is considered contaminated once neck of ampule has been placed on a nonsterile surface.
- *You inject air into inverted ampule, spraying medication:* Wash hands to remove any medication. If any medication has gotten into eyes, perform eye irrigation. Obtain a new ampule for medication dose. Report injury, if appropriate, according to facility policy.
- *Plunger becomes contaminated before inserted into ampule:* Discard needle and syringe and start over. If plunger is contaminated after medication is drawn into the syringe, it is not necessary to discard and start over. The contaminated plunger will enter the barrel of the syringe when pushing the medication out and will not come in contact with the medication and will not contaminate the medication.

SPECIAL CONSIDERATIONS

- When mixing medications in one syringe, preparation of medications in one syringe depends on how the medication is supplied. When preparing medications from an ampule and a vial, prepare the medication in the vial first. Draw up the medication in the ampule after the medication in the vial.

Skill 4 ▶ Removing Medication From a Vial

A **vial** is a glass bottle with a self-sealing stopper through which medication is removed. For safety in transporting and storing, the vial top is usually covered with a metal or plastic cap that can be removed easily. The self-sealing stopper that is then exposed is the means of entrance into the vial. Single-dose vials are used once, and then discarded, regardless of the amount of the drug that is used from the vial. Multidose vials contain several doses of medication and can be used multiple times. The Centers for Disease Control and Prevention (CDC) recommends that medications packaged as multiuse vials be assigned to a single patient whenever possible (CDC, n.d.b). In addition, it is recommended that the top of the vial be cleaned before each entry, and that a new sterile needle and syringe are used for each entry (CDC, 2011).

The medication contained in a vial can be in liquid or powder form. Powdered forms must be dissolved in an appropriate diluent before administration. The following skill reviews removing liquid medication from a vial. Refer to the accompanying Skill Variation for steps to reconstitute powdered medication.

DELEGATION CONSIDERATIONS	The preparation of medication from a vial is not delegated to nursing assistive personnel (NAP) or to unlicensed assistive personnel (UAP). Depending on the state's nurse practice act and the organization's policies and procedures, the preparation of medication from a vial may be delegated to licensed practical/vocational nurses (LPN/LVNs). The decision to delegate must be based on careful analysis of the patient's needs and circumstances, as well as the qualifications of the person to whom the task is being delegated.

EQUIPMENT

- Sterile syringe and needle or blunt cannula (size depends on medication being administered)
- Vial of medication
- Antimicrobial swab
- Second needle (optional)
- Filter needle (optional)
- Electronic Medication Administration Record (eMAR) or Medication Administration Record (MAR)

ASSESSMENT	Assess the appropriateness of the drug for the patient. Review assessment and laboratory data that may influence drug administration. Assess the medication in the vial for any discoloration or particles. Check expiration date before administering medication. Verify patient name, dose, route, and time of administration.

NURSING DIAGNOSIS

Determine related factors for the nursing diagnoses based on the patient's current status. Appropriate nursing diagnoses include:

- Risk for infection
- Deficient knowledge
- Risk for injury

OUTCOME IDENTIFICATION AND PLANNING	The expected outcome to achieve when removing medication from a vial is withdrawal of the medication into a syringe in a sterile manner; the medication is free from contamination; and the proper dose is prepared.

IMPLEMENTATION

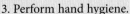

ACTION	RATIONALE
1. Gather equipment. Check the medication order against the original order in the medical record, according to facility policy. Clarify any inconsistencies. Check the patient's health record for allergies.	This comparison helps to identify errors that may have occurred when orders were transcribed. The primary care provider's order or prescription is the legal record of medication orders for each facility.
2. Know the actions, special nursing considerations, safe dose ranges, purpose of administration, and adverse effects of the medications to be administered. Consider the appropriateness of the medication for this patient.	This knowledge aids the nurse in evaluating the therapeutic effect of the medication in relation to the patient's disorder and can also be used to educate the patient about the medication.
3. Perform hand hygiene.	Hand hygiene deters the spread of microorganisms.
4. Move the medication supply system to the outside of the patient's room or prepare for administration at the medication supply system in the medication area. Alternatively, access the medication administration supply system at or inside the patient's room.	Organization facilitates error-free administration and saves time.

(continued)

Skill 4 ▶ Removing Medication From a Vial *(continued)*

ACTION	RATIONALE
5. Unlock the medication supply system or drawer. Enter pass code and scan employee identification, if required.	Locking the medication supply system or drawer safeguards each patient's medication supply. Facility accrediting organizations require medication supply systems to be locked when not in use. Entering pass code and scanning ID allows only authorized users into the system and identifies the user for documentation by the computer.
6. **Prepare medications for one patient at a time.**	This prevents errors in medication administration.
7. Read the eMAR/MAR and select the proper medication from the medication supply system or the patient's medication drawer.	This is the *first* check of the label.
8. Compare the label with the eMAR/MAR. Check expiration dates and perform calculations, if necessary. Scan the bar code on the package, if required.	This is the *second* check of the label. Verify calculations with another nurse to ensure safety, if necessary.
9. Remove the metal or plastic cap on the vial that protects the self-sealing stopper.	Cap needs to be removed to access medication in the vial.
10. **Scrub the self-sealing stopper top with the antimicrobial swab and allow to dry.**	Antimicrobial swab removes surface microbial contamination. Allowing the antimicrobial solution to dry completely (15 to 30 seconds) ensures complete antimicrobial effectiveness (Harper, 2014). Drying also prevents antimicrobial solution from entering the vial on the needle.
11. Remove the cap from the needle or blunt cannula by pulling it straight off. **If the vial in use is a multidose vial,** touch the plunger only at the knob and draw back an amount of air into the syringe that is equal to the specific dose of medication to be withdrawn. If the vial in use is a single-use vial, there is no need to draw air into the syringe.	Pulling the cap off in a straight manner prevents accidental needlestick injury. Handling the plunger only at the knob will keep the shaft of the plunger sterile. Because a vial is a sealed container, injection of an equal amount of air (before fluid is removed) is required to prevent the formation of a partial vacuum. If not enough air is injected, the negative pressure makes it difficult to withdraw the medication after repeated use.
12. Hold the vial on a flat surface. Pierce the self-sealing stopper in the center with the needle tip and inject the measured air into the space above the solution (Figure 1). **Do not inject air into the solution.** If the vial in use is a single-use vial, there is no need to inject air into the vial.	Air bubbled through the solution could result in withdrawal of an inaccurate amount of medication.

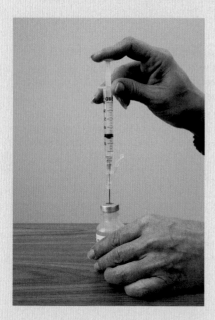

FIGURE 1. Injecting air with vial upright.

ACTION

RATIONALE

13. Invert the vial. **Keep the tip of the needle or blunt cannula below the fluid level (Figure 2).**

This prevents air from being aspirated into the syringe.

14. Hold the vial in one hand and use the other to withdraw the medication. **Touch the plunger only at the knob. Draw up the prescribed amount of medication while holding the syringe vertically and at eye level (Figure 3).**

Handling the plunger only at the knob will keep the shaft of the plunger sterile. Holding the syringe at eye level facilitates accurate reading, and the vertical position makes removal of air bubbles from the syringe easy.

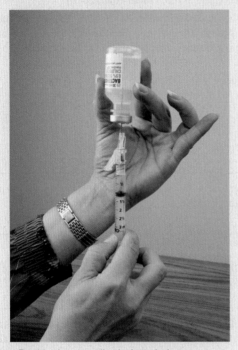

FIGURE 2. Positioning needle tip in solution.

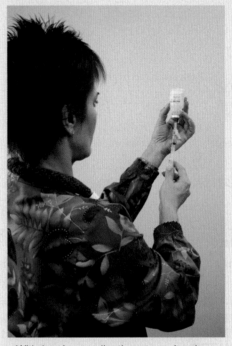

FIGURE 3. Withdrawing medication at eye level.

15. If any air bubbles accumulate in the syringe, tap the barrel of the syringe sharply and move the needle past the fluid into the air space to re-inject the air bubble into the vial. Return the needle tip to the solution and continue withdrawal of the medication.

Removal of air bubbles is necessary to ensure an accurate dose of medication.

16. After the correct dose is withdrawn, remove the needle from the vial and carefully replace the cap over the needle. Some facilities require changing the needle, if one was used to withdraw the medication, before administering the medication.

Capping prevents contamination of the needle and protects against accidental needlesticks. A one-handed recap method may be used as long as care is taken not to contaminate the needle during the process. Changing the needle may be necessary because passing the needle through the stopper on the vial may dull the needle. In addition, it ensures the tip of the needle is free from medication residue, significantly reducing pain intensity associated with the injection (Ağaç & Günes, 2010).

17. **Check the amount of medication in the syringe with the medication dose and discard any surplus.**

Careful measurement ensures that the correct dose is withdrawn.

18. **Depending on facility policy, the third check of the label may occur at this point. If so, when all medications for one patient have been prepared, recheck the labels with the eMAR/MAR before taking the medications to the patient. However, many facilities require the third check to occur at the bedside, after identifying the patient.**

This *third* check ensures accuracy and helps to prevent errors. *Note:* Many facilities require the *third* check to occur at the bedside, after identifying the patient and before administration.

(continued)

Skill 4 ▶ Removing Medication From a Vial *(continued)*

ACTION	**RATIONALE**
19. If a multidose vial is being used, label the vial with the date and time opened and the beyond-use date (see Special Considerations), and store the vial containing the remaining medication according to facility policy. Limit the use of multiple-dose vials and dedicate them to a single patient whenever possible (CDC, n.d.b).	Because the vial is sealed, the medication inside remains sterile and can be used for future injections. Labeling the opened vials with a date, time, and beyond-use date limits its use after a specific time period. Limiting use of multiple-dose vials and dedicating their use to a single patient when possible limits risk of contamination and transfer of microorganisms (CDC, n.d.b; Dolan et al., 2016).
20. Lock the medication supply system before leaving it.	Locking the medication supply system or drawer safeguards the patient's medication supply. Facility accrediting organizations require medication supply systems to be locked when not in use.
21. Perform hand hygiene.	Hand hygiene deters the spread of microorganisms.
22. Proceed with administration, based on prescribed route.	See appropriate skill for prescribed route.

EVALUATION

The expected outcomes have been met when the medication was withdrawn into the syringe in a sterile manner and is free from contamination, and the proper dose is prepared.

DOCUMENTATION

Guidelines

It is not necessary to record the removal of the medication from a vial. Prompt recording of administration of the medication is required immediately after it is administered.

UNEXPECTED SITUATIONS AND ASSOCIATED INTERVENTIONS

- *A piece of self-sealing stopper is noticed floating in the medication in the syringe:* Discard the syringe, needle, and vial. Obtain a new vial, syringe, and needle and prepare dose as ordered.
- *As the needle attached to the syringe filled with air is inserted into vial, the plunger is immediately pulled down:* If possible to withdraw medication, continue steps as explained above. If such a vacuum has formed that this is impossible, remove syringe and inject more air into the vial.
- *Plunger is contaminated before injecting air into vial:* Discard needle and syringe and start over.
- *Plunger is contaminated after medication is drawn into syringe:* It is not necessary to discard needle and syringe and start over. The contaminated plunger will enter the barrel of the syringe when pushing the medication out and will not come in contact with the medication, and therefore will not contaminate the medication.

SPECIAL CONSIDERATIONS

- When mixing medications in one syringe, preparation of medications in one syringe depends on how the medication is supplied. When using a single-dose vial and a multidose vial, inject air into the multidose vial and draw the medication in the multidose vial into the syringe first. This prevents the contents of the multidose vial from being contaminated with the medication in the single-dose vial. The steps to follow when preparing medications from two multidose vials in one syringe are outlined in Skill 5.
- Vials used to draw two or more medications into a single syringe must be discarded after use (Dolan et al., 2016).
- Do not administer medication from a single-dose vial to multiple patients (CDC, n.d.b).
- Limit the use of multiple-dose vials and dedicate them to a single patient whenever possible (CDC, n.d.b).
- Multiple-dose vials must be labeled with a beyond-use date when first opened, as indicated by facility policy (Dolan et al., 2016).

Skill Variation ▶ Reconstituting Powdered Medication in a Vial

Drugs that are unstable in liquid form are often provided in a dry powder form. The powder must be mixed with the correct amount of appropriate solution (diluent) to prepare the medication for administration. Verify the correct amount and correct solution type for the specific medication prescribed. This information is found on the vial label, package insert, in a drug reference, an on-line pharmacy source, or from the pharmacist. To reconstitute powdered medication:

1. Gather equipment. Check the medication order against the original order in the medical record, according to facility policy.
2. Know the actions, special nursing considerations, safe dose ranges, purpose of administration, and adverse effects of the medications to be administered. Consider the appropriateness of the medication for this patient.
   3. Perform hand hygiene.

4. Move the medication supply system to the outside of the patient's room or prepare for administration at the medication supply system in the medication area. Alternatively, access the medication administration supply system at or inside the patient's room.
5. Unlock the medication supply system or drawer. Enter pass code and scan employee identification, if required.
6. **Prepare medications for one patient at a time.**
7. Read the eMAR/MAR and select the proper medication and diluent from medication supply system or from the patient's medication drawer. This is the *first* check of the medication label.
8. Compare the labels with the eMAR/MAR. This is the *second* check of the medication label. Check expiration dates and perform calculations, check medication calculation with another nurse. Scan the bar code on the package, if required.

9. Remove the metal or plastic cap on the medication vial and diluent vial that protects the self-sealing stoppers.
10. Scrub the self-sealing tops on both the diluent and powdered medication vials with the antimicrobial swab and allow to dry.
11. **Draw up the appropriate amount of diluent into the syringe.**
12. Insert the needle or blunt cannula through the center of the self-sealing stopper on the powdered medication vial.
13. Inject the diluent into the powdered medication vial.
14. Remove the needle or blunt cannula from the vial and replace cap.
15. **Gently agitate the vial to mix the powdered medication and the diluent completely. Do not shake the vial.**
16. **Draw up the prescribed amount of medication while holding the syringe vertically and at eye level.**
17. After the correct dose is withdrawn, remove the needle from the vial and carefully replace the cap over the needle. Some facilities require changing the needle, if one was used to withdraw the medication, before administering the medication.
18. **Check the amount of medication in the syringe with the medication dose and discard any surplus.**
19. **Depending on facility policy, the *third* check of the label may occur at this point. If so, recheck the label with the eMAR/MAR before taking the medications to the patient. However, many facilities require the third check to occur at the bedside, after identifying the patient.**
20. **Lock the medication supply system before leaving it.**
    21. Perform hand hygiene.

22. Proceed with administration, based on prescribed route.

Skill 5 ▶ Mixing Medications From Two Vials in One Syringe

Preparation of medications in one syringe depends on how the medication is supplied. When using two multidose vials, air is injected into both vials before withdrawing the first medication, to prevent the accidental injection of medication into the second vial. When using a single-dose vial and a multidose vial, air is injected into the multidose vial and the medication in the multidose vial is drawn into the syringe first. This prevents the contents of the multidose vial from being contaminated with the medication in the single-dose vial. The CDC recommends that medications packaged as multiuse vials be assigned to a single patient whenever possible (CDC, n.d.b). In addition, it is recommended that the top of the vial be cleaned before each entry, and that a new sterile needle and syringe are used before each entry (CDC, 2011).

(continued)

Skill 5 ▶ Mixing Medications From Two Vials in One Syringe *(continued)*

When considering mixing two medications in one syringe, you must ensure that the two drugs are compatible. Be aware of drug incompatibilities when preparing medications in one syringe. Certain medications are incompatible with other drugs in the same syringe. Other drugs have limited compatibility and should be administered within 15 minutes of preparation. Mixing more than two drugs in one syringe is not recommended. If it must be done, contact the pharmacist to determine the compatibility of the three drugs, as well as the compatibility of their pH values and the preservatives that may be present in each drug. A drug-compatibility table should be available to nurses who are preparing medications.

Insulin, with many types available for use, is an example of a medication that may be combined together in one syringe for injection. Insulins vary in their onset and duration of action and are classified as rapid acting, short acting, intermediate acting, and long acting (Frandsen & Pennington, 2014). Before administering any insulin, be aware of the onset time, peak, and duration of effects, and ensure that proper food is available. Be aware that some insulins, such as glargine and detemir, cannot be mixed with other insulins. Refer to a drug reference for a listing of the different types of insulin and action specific to each type.

Insulin is used as the sample medication in the steps outlined below for mixing two medications in one syringe. Insulin is typically available in multidose vials, and dosages are calculated in units. The scale commonly used is U100, which is based on 100 units of insulin contained in 1 mL of solution. An insulin syringe is also calibrated in units. Insulin is also available in injection pens, which eliminate the need to prepare two medications in one syringe. Insulin injection pens are prefilled devices that combine the insulin container and syringe. Patients attach a needle for each administration, dial a dose of insulin, and depress a plunger to administer the dose. Use of an insulin injection pen is outlined in the Skill Variation in Skill 7 on page 33.

DELEGATION CONSIDERATIONS	The preparation of medication from two vials is not delegated to nursing assistive personnel (NAP) or to unlicensed assistive personnel (UAP). Depending on the state's nurse practice act and the organization's policies and procedures, the preparation of medication from two vials may be delegated to licensed practical/vocational nurses (LPN/LVNs). The decision to delegate must be based on careful analysis of the patient's needs and circumstances, as well as the qualifications of the person to whom the task is being delegated.
EQUIPMENT	The preparation of two types of insulin in one syringe is used as the example in the following procedure. • Two vials of medication (insulin in this example) • Sterile syringe (insulin syringe in this example) • Antimicrobial swabs • Electronic Medication Administration Record (eMAR) or Medication Administration Record (MAR)
ASSESSMENT	Assess the appropriateness of the drug for the patient. Review medical history, allergy, assessment, and laboratory data that may influence drug administration. Determine the compatibility of the two medications. Not all insulin can be mixed together. Assess the contents of each vial of insulin. It is very important to be familiar with the particular drug's properties to be able to assess the quality of the medication in the vial before withdrawal. Unmodified preparations of insulin typically appear as clear substances, so they should be without particles or foreign matter. Modified preparations of insulin are typically suspensions, so they do not appear as clear substances. Check the expiration date before administering the medication. Check the patient's blood glucose level, if appropriate, before administering the insulin. Verify patient name, dose, route, and time of administration.
NURSING DIAGNOSIS	Determine related factors for the nursing diagnoses based on the patient's current status. Appropriate nursing diagnoses include: • Risk for infection • Deficient knowledge • Risk for unstable blood glucose level

IMPLEMENTATION

ACTION	RATIONALE
1. Gather equipment. Check medication order against the original order in the medical record, according to facility policy.	This comparison helps to identify errors that may have occurred when orders were transcribed. The primary care provider's order or prescription is the legal record of medication orders for each facility.
2. Know the actions, special nursing considerations, safe dose ranges, purpose of administration, and adverse effects of the medications to be administered. Consider the appropriateness of the medication for this patient.	This knowledge aids the nurse in evaluating the therapeutic effect of the medication in relation to the patient's disorder and can also be used to educate the patient about the medication.
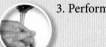 3. Perform hand hygiene.	Hand hygiene prevents the spread of microorganisms.
4. Move the medication supply system to the outside of the patient's room or prepare for administration at the medication supply system in the medication area. Alternatively, access the medication administration supply system at or inside the patient's room.	Organization facilitates error-free administration and saves time.
5. Unlock the medication supply system or drawer. Enter pass code and scan employee identification, if required.	Locking the supply system or drawer safeguards each patient's medication supply. Facility accrediting organizations require medication supply systems to be locked when not in use. Entering pass code and scanning ID allows only authorized users into the system and identifies the user for documentation by the computer.
6. **Prepare medications for one patient at a time.**	This prevents errors in medication administration.
7. Read the eMAR/MAR and select the proper medications from the medication supply system or the patient's medication drawer.	This is the *first* check of the label.
8. Compare the labels with the eMAR/MAR. Check expiration dates and perform dosage calculations, if necessary. Scan the bar code on the package, if required.	This is the *second* check of the labels. Verify calculations with another nurse to ensure safety, if necessary.
9. If necessary, remove the cap that protects the self-sealing stopper on each vial.	The cap protects the self-sealing top.
10. **If medication is a suspension (e.g., a modified insulin, such as NPH insulin), roll and agitate the vial to mix it well.**	There is controversy regarding how to mix insulin in suspension. Some sources advise rolling the vial; others advise shaking the vial. Consult facility policy. Regardless of the method used, it is essential that the suspension be mixed well to avoid administering an inconsistent dose.
11. **Scrub the self-sealing stopper top with the antimicrobial swab and allow to dry.**	Antimicrobial swab removes surface microbial contamination. Allowing the antimicrobial solution to dry completely (15 to 30 seconds) ensures complete antimicrobial effectiveness (Harper, 2014). Drying also prevents antimicrobial solution from entering the vial on the needle.
12. Remove cap from needle by pulling it straight off. Touch the plunger only at the knob. Draw back an amount of air into the syringe that is equal to the dose of modified insulin to be withdrawn.	Pulling the cap off in a straight manner prevents accidental needlestick. Handling the plunger only by the knob ensures sterility of the shaft of the plunger. Before fluid is removed, injection of an equal amount of air is required to prevent the formation of a partial vacuum, because a vial is a sealed container. If not enough air is injected, the negative pressure makes it difficult to withdraw the medication with repeated use.

(continued)

Skill 5 ▶ Mixing Medications From Two Vials in One Syringe *(continued)*

13. Hold the modified vial on a flat surface. Pierce the self-sealing stopper in the center with the needle tip and inject the measured air into the space above the solution (Figure 1). Do not inject air into the solution. Withdraw the needle.

14. Draw back an amount of air into the syringe that is equal to the dose of unmodified insulin to be withdrawn.

15. Hold the unmodified vial on a flat surface. Pierce the self-sealing stopper in the center with the needle tip and inject the measured air into the space above the solution (Figure 2). Do not inject air into the solution. Keep the needle in the vial.

Unmodified insulin should never be contaminated with modified insulin. Placing air in the modified insulin first without allowing the needle to contact the insulin ensures that the second vial-entered (unmodified) insulin is not contaminated by the medication in the other vial. Air bubbled through the solution could result in withdrawal of an inaccurate amount of medication.

A vial is a sealed container. Therefore, injection of an equal amount of air (before fluid is removed) is required to prevent the formation of a partial vacuum. If not enough air is injected, the negative pressure makes it difficult to withdraw the medication.

Air bubbled through the solution could result in withdrawal of an inaccurate amount of medication.

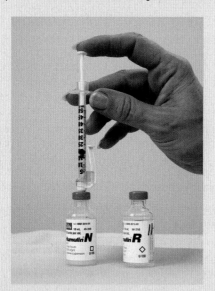

FIGURE 1. Injecting air into modified insulin preparation.

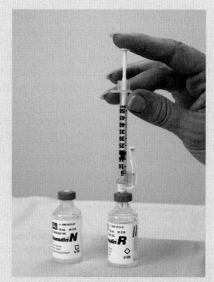

FIGURE 2. Injecting air into unmodified insulin vial.

16. Invert the vial of unmodified insulin. Hold the vial in one hand and use the other to withdraw the medication. **Touch the plunger only at the knob. Draw up the prescribed amount of medication while holding the syringe at eye level and vertically (Figure 3).** Turn the vial over and then remove the needle from the vial.

17. Check that there are no air bubbles in the syringe.

18. **Check the amount of medication in the syringe with the medication dose and discard any surplus.**

19. **Recheck the vial label with the eMAR/MAR.**

20. Calculate the endpoint on the syringe for the combined insulin amount by adding the number of units for each dose together.

Holding the syringe at eye level facilitates accurate reading, and the vertical position allows easy removal of air bubbles from the syringe. First dose is prepared and is not contaminated by insulin that contains modifiers.

The presence of air in the syringe would result in an inaccurate dose of medication.

Careful measurement ensures that correct dose is withdrawn.

This is the *third* check to ensure accuracy and to prevent errors. It must be checked now for the first medication in the syringe, as it is not possible to ensure accuracy once a second drug is in the syringe.

Allows for accurate withdrawal of the second dose.

ACTION	RATIONALE

21. Insert the needle into the modified vial and invert it, taking care not to push the plunger and inject medication from the syringe into the vial. Invert vial of modified insulin. Hold the vial in one hand and use the other to withdraw the medication. **Touch the plunger only at the knob. Draw up the prescribed amount of medication while holding the syringe at eye level and vertically (Figure 4). Take care to withdraw only the prescribed amount.** Turn the vial over and then remove the needle from the vial. Carefully recap the needle. Carefully replace the cap over the needle.

Previous addition of air eliminates need to create positive pressure. Holding the syringe at eye level facilitates accurate reading. Capping the needle prevents contamination and protects the nurse against accidental needlesticks. A one-handed recap method may be used as long as care is taken to ensure that the needle remains sterile.

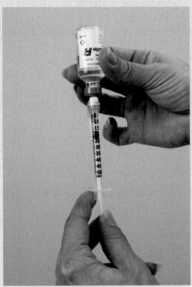

FIGURE 3. Withdrawing prescribed amount of unmodified insulin.

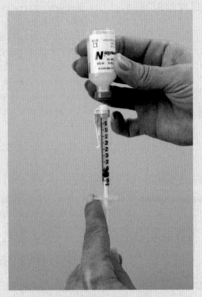

FIGURE 4. Withdrawing modified insulin.

22. **Check the amount of medication in the syringe with the medication dose.**

Careful measurement ensures that correct dose is withdrawn.

23. **Depending on facility policy, the third check of the label may occur at this point. If so, recheck the label with the MAR before taking the medications to the patient. However, many facilities require the third check to occur at the bedside, after identifying the patient.**

This *third* check ensures accuracy and helps to prevent errors. *Note:* Many facilities require the *third* check to occur at the bedside, after identifying the patient and before administration.

24. **Label the vials with the date and time opened and beyond-use date, and store the vials containing the remaining medication, according to facility policy.**

Because the vial is sealed, the medication inside remains sterile and can be used for future injections. Labeling the opened vials with a date and time limits its use after a specific time period. The CDC recommends that medications packaged as multiuse vials be assigned to a single patient whenever possible (CDC, n.d.b; Dolan et al., 2016).

25. **Lock the medication supply system before leaving it.**

Locking the medication supply system or drawer safeguards the patient's medication supply. Facility accrediting organizations require medication supply systems to be locked when not in use.

26. Perform hand hygiene.

Hand hygiene deters the spread of microorganisms.

27. Proceed with administration, based on prescribed route.

See appropriate skill for prescribed route.

(*continued*)

Skill 5 ▶ Mixing Medications From Two Vials in One Syringe *(continued)*

EVALUATION	The expected outcomes have been met when the medication is withdrawn into the syringe in a sterile manner and is free from contamination and the proper dose is prepared.

DOCUMENTATION

Guidelines

It is not necessary to record the removal of the medication from the vials. Prompt recording of administration of the medication is required immediately after it is administered.

UNEXPECTED SITUATIONS AND ASSOCIATED INTERVENTIONS

- *You contaminate the plunger before injecting air into the insulin vial:* Discard the needle and syringe and start over.
- *The plunger is contaminated after medication is drawn into the syringe:* It is not necessary to discard and start over. The contaminated plunger will enter the barrel of the syringe when pushing the medication out and will not contaminate the medication.
- *You allow modified insulin to come in contact with the needle before entering the unmodified insulin vial:* Discard needle and syringe and start over.
- *You notice that the combined amount is not the ordered amount (e.g., you have less or more units in combined syringe than ordered):* Discard syringe and start over. There is no way to know for sure which dosage is wrong or which medication should be expelled.
- *You inject medication from the first vial (in syringe) into the second vial:* Discard vial and syringe and start over.

SPECIAL CONSIDERATIONS

General Considerations

- A patient with diabetes who is visually impaired may find it helpful to use a magnifying apparatus that fits around the syringe.
- Before attempting to explain or demonstrate devices that help low-vision diabetic patients to prepare their medication, attempt to use the device yourself under similar circumstances. To detect any difficulties the patient may experience, practice using the aid with your eyes closed or in a poorly lit room.

Infant and Child Considerations

- School-age children are generally able to prepare and administer their own injections, such as insulin, with supervision (Kyle & Carman, 2017). Parents/significant others and the child should be involved in teaching.

Skill 6 ▶ Administering an Intradermal Injection

Intradermal injections are administered into the dermis, just below the epidermis. The intradermal route has the longest absorption time of all parenteral routes. For this reason, intradermal injections are used for sensitivity tests, such as tuberculin and allergy tests, and local anesthesia. The advantage of the intradermal route for these tests is that the body's reaction to substances is easily visible, and degrees of reaction are discernible by comparative study.

Sites commonly used are the inner surface of the forearm and the upper back, under the scapula. Equipment used for an intradermal injection includes a tuberculin syringe calibrated in tenths and hundredths of a milliliter and a 0.25- to 0.5-in, 25- or 27-gauge needle. The dosage given intradermally is small, usually less than 0.5 mL. The angle of administration for an intradermal injection is 5 to 15 degrees.

DELEGATION CONSIDERATIONS

The administration of an intradermal injection is not delegated to nursing assistive personnel (NAP) or to unlicensed assistive personnel (UAP). Depending on the state's nurse practice act and the organization's policies and procedures, the administration of an intradermal injection may be delegated to licensed practical/vocational nurses (LPN/LVNs). The decision to delegate must be based on careful analysis of the patient's needs and circumstances, as well as the qualifications of the person to whom the task is being delegated.

EQUIPMENT

- Prescribed medication
- Sterile syringe, usually a tuberculin syringe calibrated in tenths and hundredths, and a needle, ¼- to ½-in, 25- or 27-gauge
- Antimicrobial swab
- Disposable gloves
- Small gauze square
- Electronic Medication Administration Record (eMAR) or Medication Administration Record (MAR)
- PPE, as indicated

ASSESSMENT

Assess the appropriateness of the drug for the patient. Review medical history, allergy, assessment, and laboratory data that may influence drug administration. Check expiration date before administering medication. Assess the site on the patient where the injection is to be given. Avoid areas of broken or open skin. Avoid areas that are highly pigmented, and those that have lesions, bruises, or scars and are hairy. Assess the patient's knowledge of the medication. This may provide an opportune time for patient education. Verify the patient's name, dose, route, and time of administration.

NURSING DIAGNOSIS

Determine related factors for the nursing diagnoses based on the patient's current status. Appropriate nursing diagnoses may include:

- Deficient knowledge
- Risk for infection
- Risk for injury

OUTCOME IDENTIFICATION AND PLANNING

The expected outcome to achieve when administering an intradermal injection is that the medication is injected and a wheal appears at the injection site. Other outcomes that may be appropriate include the following: the patient refrains from rubbing the site; the patient does not experience adverse effects; and the patient understands and complies with the medication regimen.

IMPLEMENTATION

ACTION	RATIONALE
1. Gather equipment. Check each medication order against the original order in the medical record according to facility policy. Clarify any inconsistencies. Check the patient's health record for allergies.	This comparison helps to identify errors that may have occurred when orders were transcribed. The primary care provider's order or prescription is the legal record of medication orders for each facility.
2. Know the actions, special nursing considerations, safe dose ranges, purpose of administration, and adverse effects of the medications to be administered. Consider the appropriateness of the medication for this patient.	This knowledge aids the nurse in evaluating the therapeutic effect of the medication in relation to the patient's disorder and can also be used to educate the patient about the medication.
3. Perform hand hygiene.	Hand hygiene deters the spread of microorganisms.
4. Move the medication supply system to the outside of the patient's room or prepare for administration at the medication supply system in the medication area. Alternatively, access the medication administration supply system at or inside the patient's room.	Organization facilitates error-free administration and saves time.
5. Unlock the medication supply system or drawer. Enter pass code and scan employee identification, if required.	Locking the medication supply system or drawer safeguards each patient's medication supply. Facility accrediting organizations require medication supply systems to be locked when not in use. Entering pass code and scanning ID allows only authorized users into the system and identifies the user for documentation by the computer.

(continued)

Skill 6 ▶ Administering an Intradermal Injection *(continued)*

ACTION	RATIONALE
6. Prepare medications for one patient at a time.	This prevents errors in medication administration.
7. Read the eMAR/MAR and select the proper medication from the medication supply system or the patient's medication drawer.	This is the *first* check of the label.
8. Compare the label with the eMAR/MAR. Check expiration dates and perform calculations, if necessary. Scan the bar code on the package, if required.	This is the *second* check of the label. Verify calculations with another nurse to ensure safety.
9. If necessary, withdraw the medication from an ampule or vial as described in Skills 3 and 4.	
10. Depending on facility policy, the third check of the label may occur at this point. If so, when all medications for one patient have been prepared, recheck the labels with the eMAR/MAR before taking the medications to the patient. However, many facilities require the third check to occur at the bedside, after identifying the patient.	This *third* check ensures accuracy and helps to prevent errors. *Note:* Many facilities require the *third* check to occur at the bedside, after identifying the patient and before administration.
11. Lock the medication supply system before leaving it.	Locking the medication supply system or drawer safeguards the patient's medication supply. Facility accrediting organizations require medication supply systems to be locked when not in use.
12. Transport medications to the patient's bedside carefully, and keep the medications in sight at all times.	Careful handling and close observation prevent accidental or deliberate disarrangement of medications.
13. Ensure that the patient receives the medications at the correct time.	Check facility policy, which may allow for administration within a period of 30 minutes before or 30 minutes after the designated time.
14. Perform hand hygiene and put on PPE, if indicated.	Hand hygiene and PPE prevent the spread of microorganisms. PPE is required based on transmission precautions.
15. Identify the patient. Compare the information with the eMAR/MAR. The patient should be identified using at least two of the following methods (The Joint Commission, 2018):	Identifying the patient ensures the right patient receives the medications and helps prevent errors. The patient's room number or physical location is not used as an identifier (The Joint Commission, 2018). Replace the identification band if it is missing or inaccurate in any way.
a. Check the name on the patient's identification band.	This requires a response from the patient, but illness and strange surroundings often cause patients to be confused.
b. Check the identification number on the patient's identification band.	
c. Check the birth date on the patient's identification band.	
d. Ask the patient to state his or her name and birth date, based on facility policy.	
16. Close the door to the room or pull the bedside curtain.	This provides patient privacy.
17. Complete necessary assessments before administering medications. Check allergy bracelet or ask the patient about allergies. Explain the purpose and action of the medication to the patient.	Assessment is a prerequisite to administration of medications. Explanation provides rationale, increases knowledge, and reduces anxiety.
18. Scan the patient's bar code on the identification band, if required.	Provides an additional check to ensure that the medication is given to the right patient.
19. Based on facility policy, the third check of the label may occur at this point. If so, recheck the labels with the eMAR/MAR before administering the medications to the patient.	Many facilities require the *third* check to occur at the bedside, after identifying the patient and before administration. If facility policy directs the *third* check at this time, this *third* check ensures accuracy and helps to prevent errors.
20. Put on clean gloves.	Gloves help prevent exposure to contaminants.

ACTION	RATIONALE
21. Select an appropriate administration site. Assist the patient to the appropriate position for the site chosen. Drape, as needed, to expose only site area to be used.	Appropriate site prevents injury and allows for accurate reading of the test site at the appropriate time. Draping provides privacy and warmth.
22. Cleanse the site with an antimicrobial swab while wiping with a firm, circular motion and moving outward from the injection site. Allow the skin to dry.	Pathogens on the skin can be forced into the tissues by the needle. Moving from the center outward prevents contamination of the site. Allowing the antimicrobial solution to dry completely (15 to 30 seconds) ensures complete antimicrobial effectiveness (Harper, 2014), and prevents introducing alcohol into the tissue, which can be irritating and uncomfortable.
23. Remove the needle cap with the nondominant hand by pulling it straight off.	This technique lessens the risk of an accidental needlestick.
24. Use the nondominant hand to spread the skin taut over the injection site (Figure 1).	Taut skin provides an easy entrance into intradermal tissue.
25. Hold the syringe in the dominant hand, between the thumb and forefinger with the bevel of the needle up.	Using the dominant hand allows for easy, appropriate handling of the syringe. Having the bevel up allows for smooth piercing of the skin and introduction of medication into the dermis.
26. Hold the syringe at a 5- to 15-degree angle from the site. Place the needle almost flat against the patient's skin (Figure 2), bevel side up, and insert the needle into the skin. Insert the needle only about ⅛ in with entire bevel under the skin.	The dermis is entered when the needle is held as nearly parallel to the skin as possible and is inserted about ⅛ in.

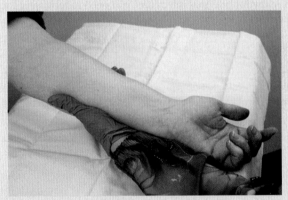

FIGURE 1. Spreading skin taut over injection site.

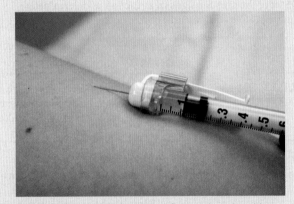

FIGURE 2. Inserting needle almost flat against the skin.

27. Once the needle is in place, steady the lower end of the syringe. Slide your dominant hand to the end of the plunger.	Prevents injury and inadvertent advancement or withdrawal of needle.
28. Slowly inject the agent while watching for a small wheal to appear (Figure 3).	The appearance of a wheal indicates the medication is in the dermis.

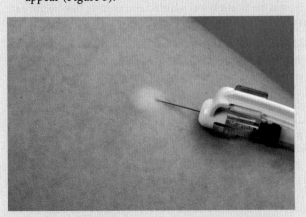

FIGURE 3. Observing for wheal while injecting medication.

(*continued*)

Skill 6 ▶ Administering an Intradermal Injection *(continued)*

ACTION	RATIONALE
29. Withdraw the needle quickly at the same angle that it was inserted. Do not recap the used needle. Engage the safety shield or needle guard.	Withdrawing the needle quickly and at the angle at which it entered the skin minimizes tissue damage and discomfort for the patient. Safety shield or needle guard prevents accidental needlestick injury.
30. **Do not massage the area after removing needle. Tell the patient not to rub or scratch the site. If necessary, gently blot the site with a dry gauze square. Do not apply pressure or rub the site.**	Massaging or rubbing the area where an intradermal injection is given may spread the medication to underlying subcutaneous tissue.
31. Assist the patient to a position of comfort.	This provides for the well-being of the patient.
32. Discard the needle and syringe in the appropriate receptacle.	Proper disposal of the needle prevents injury.
33. Remove gloves and additional PPE, if used. Perform hand hygiene.	Proper removal of PPE reduces the risk for infection transmission and contamination of other items. Hand hygiene prevents the spread of microorganisms.
34. Document the administration of the medication immediately after administration. See Documentation section below.	Timely documentation helps to ensure patient safety.
35. Evaluate the patient's response to the medication within the appropriate time frame.	The patient needs to be evaluated for therapeutic and adverse effects from the medication.
36. Observe the area for signs of a reaction at determined intervals after administration. Inform the patient of the need for inspection.	With many intradermal injections, you need to look for a localized reaction in the area of the injection at the appropriate interval(s) determined by the type of medication and purpose. Explaining this to the patient increases compliance.

EVALUATION	The expected outcomes have been met when you note a wheal at the injection site; the patient refrains from rubbing the site; the patient did not experience adverse effects; and the patient verbalizes an understanding of, and complies with, the medication regimen.
DOCUMENTATION *Guidelines*	Record each medication administered on the eMAR/MAR or health record using the required format, including date, time, and the site of administration, immediately after administration. Some facilities recommend circling the injection site with ink. Circling the injection site easily identifies the intradermal injection site and allows for future careful observation of the exact area. If using a bar-code system, medication administration is automatically recorded when the bar code is scanned. PRN medications require documentation of the reason for administration. Prompt recording avoids the possibility of accidentally repeating the administration of the drug. If the drug was refused or omitted, record this in the appropriate area on the medication record and notify the primary care provider. This verifies the reason medication was omitted and ensures that health care personnel providing care for the patient are aware of the occurrence.
UNEXPECTED SITUATIONS AND ASSOCIATED INTERVENTIONS	• *You do not note a wheal or blister at the injection site:* Medication has been injected subcutaneously. Document according to facility policy and inform the primary care provider. You may need to obtain an order to repeat the procedure. • *Medication leaks out of the injection site before the needle is withdrawn:* Needle was inserted less than ⅛ in. Document according to facility policy and inform the primary care provider. You may need to obtain an order to repeat the procedure. • *You stick yourself with the needle before injection:* Discard needle and syringe appropriately. Follow facility policy regarding needlestick injury. Prepare new syringe with medication and administer to patient. Complete appropriate paperwork and follow facility's policy regarding accidental needlestick injuries. • *You stick yourself with the needle after injection:* Discard needle and syringe appropriately. Follow facility policy regarding needlestick injury. Complete appropriate paperwork and follow facility's policy regarding accidental needlestick injuries.

SPECIAL CONSIDERATIONS

- Fluzone Intradermal is the only vaccine in the United States administered by the intradermal route and is available for patients 18 to 64 years of age (CDC, 2015a; Sanofi Pasteur, 2016). The site of administration for this vaccine is the deltoid region of the upper arm, and the needle is inserted perpendicular to the skin (CDC, 2015a). **This vaccine should not be administered into the forearm or other site used to administer other intradermal medications.** The prefilled microinjection syringe administers a 0.1-mL dose into the dermal layer of the skin via a 30-gauge, 1.5-mL microneedle (CDC, 2015a). **No other influenza vaccine formulations should be administered by the intradermal route** (CDC, 2015a). Follow manufacturer directions for appropriate administration.
- Ongoing assessment is an important part of nursing care for both evaluation of patient response to administered medications and early detection of adverse reactions. If an adverse effect is suspected, withhold further medication doses and notify the patient's primary care provider. Additional intervention is based on type of reaction and patient assessment.
- Some facilities recommend administering intradermal injections with the bevel down instead of the bevel up. Check facility policy.

Skill 7 ▶ Administering a Subcutaneous Injection

Subcutaneous injections are administered into the adipose tissue layer just below the epidermis and dermis. This tissue has few blood vessels, so drugs administered here have a slow, sustained rate of absorption into the capillaries. Various sites may be used for subcutaneous injections, including the outer aspect of the upper arm, the abdomen (from below the costal margin to the iliac crests), the anterior aspects of the thigh, the upper back, and the upper ventral- or dorsogluteal area. Figure 1 displays the sites on the body where subcutaneous injections can be given. Absorption rates differ among the various sites. Injections in the abdomen are absorbed most rapidly; ones in the arms are absorbed somewhat more slowly; those in the thighs, even more slowly; and those in the ventral or dorsogluteal areas have the slowest absorption (American Diabetes Association [ADA], 2015).

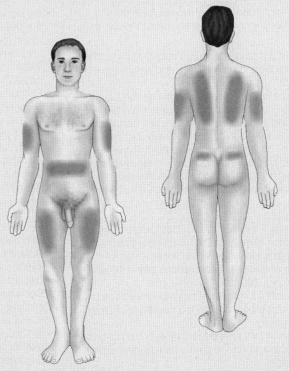

FIGURE 1. Body sites where subcutaneous injections can be given.

(continued)

Skill 7 ▶ Administering a Subcutaneous Injection *(continued)*

It is important to choose the right equipment to ensure depositing the medication into the intended subcutaneous tissue and not the underlying muscle. Equipment used for a subcutaneous injection includes a syringe of appropriate volume for the amount of drug being administered. An insulin injection pen may be used for subcutaneous injection of insulin (see the accompanying Skill Variation for technique). A 25- to 30-gauge, ⅜- to 1-in needle can be used; ⅜- and ⅝-in needles are most commonly used for subcutaneous injections. Choose the needle length based on the amount of subcutaneous tissue present, which is based on the patient's body weight and build (Annersten & Willman, 2005). Some medications are packaged in prefilled cartridges with a needle attached. Confirm that the provided needle is appropriate for the patient before use. If not, the medication will have to be transferred to another syringe and the appropriate needle attached.

Subcutaneous injections are administered at a 45- or 90-degree angle, with the 45-degree angle used only for patients with a limited amount of subcutaneous tissue. Choose the angle of needle insertion based on the amount of subcutaneous tissue present and the length of the needle. In general, insert the shorter, ⅜-in needle, at a 90-degree angle (common on prefilled and insulin syringes). The longer, ⅝-in needle, may be inserted at a 45-degree angle. The angles of insertion for subcutaneous injections.

Recommendations differ regarding pinching a skin fold for administration. Forming a skin fold is advised for thinner patients and when a longer needle is used to lift the adipose tissue away from underlying muscle and tissue. If pinching to form a skin fold is used, once the needle is inserted, release the skin and stabilize the base of the needle to avoid injecting into the compressed tissue.

Usually, no more than 1 mL of solution is given subcutaneously. Giving larger amounts adds to the patient's discomfort and may predispose to poor absorption. It is necessary to rotate sites or areas for injection if the patient is to receive frequent injections. This helps to prevent buildup of fibrous tissue and permits complete absorption of the medication. Further information regarding insulin administration and rotation of injection sites can be found in the General Considerations at the end of this skill.

Box 7-1 discusses techniques for reducing discomfort when injecting medications subcutaneously or intramuscularly.

Box 7-1 Reducing Discomfort in Subcutaneous and Intramuscular Administrations

The following are recommended techniques for reducing discomfort when injecting medications subcutaneously or intramuscularly:

• Select a needle of the smallest gauge that is appropriate for the site and solution to be injected, and select the correct needle length.
• Be sure the needle is free of medication that may irritate superficial tissues as the needle is inserted. The recommended procedure is to use two needles—one to remove the medication from the vial or ampule and a second one to inject the medication. If medication is in a prefilled syringe with a nonremovable needle and has dripped back on the needle during preparation, gently tap the barrel to remove the excess solution.
• Apply manual pressure at the insertion site by pressing the insertion site firmly for 10 seconds before needle insertion. This action stimulates the surrounding nerve endings, leading to a reduction in the sensory input from the injection and resulting decreased pain intensity (Chung, Ng, & Wong, 2002).
• Use the Z-track technique for intramuscular injections to prevent leakage of medication into the needle track, thus minimizing discomfort.
• Inject the medication into relaxed muscles. More pressure and discomfort occur when the medication is injected into a contracted muscle.

• Do not inject areas that feel hard on palpation or tender to the patient.
• Insert the needle with a dart-like motion without hesitation, and remove it quickly at the same angle at which it was inserted. These techniques reduce discomfort and tissue irritation.
• Do not administer more solution in one injection than is recommended for the site. Injecting more solution creates excess pressure in the area and increases discomfort.
• Inject the solution slowly so that it may be dispersed more easily into the surrounding tissue (10 seconds per 1 mL).
• Apply gentle pressure after injection, unless this technique is contraindicated.
• Allow the patient who is fearful of injections to talk about his or her fears. Answer the patient's questions truthfully, and explain the nature and purpose of the injection. Taking the time to offer support often allays fears and decreases discomfort.
• Rotate sites when the patient is to receive repeated injections. Injections in the same site may cause undue discomfort, irritation, or abscesses in tissues.
• Consider nonpharmacologic methods for infants and children, such as breastfeeding, the administration of sweet solutions, front-to-front upright holding, rapid injection without aspiration, administration of the most painful vaccine last, tactile stimulation, and other distractions (Harrison et al., 2014; Taddio et al., 2010).

DELEGATION CONSIDERATIONS	The administration of a subcutaneous injection is not delegated to nursing assistive personnel (NAP) or to unlicensed assistive personnel (UAP). Depending on the state's nurse practice act and the organization's policies and procedures, the administration of a subcutaneous injection may be delegated to licensed practical/vocational nurses (LPN/LVNs). The decision to delegate must be based on careful analysis of the patient's needs and circumstances, as well as the qualifications of the person to whom the task is being delegated.

EQUIPMENT	• Prescribed medication • Sterile syringe and needle. Needle size depends on the medication to be administered and patient body type (see previous discussion). • Antimicrobial swab • Nonlatex, disposable gloves • Small gauze square • Electronic Medication Administration Record (eMAR) or Medication Administration Record (MAR) • PPE, as indicated

ASSESSMENT	Assess the appropriateness of the drug for the patient. Review medical history, allergy, assessment, and laboratory data that may influence drug administration. Check expiration date before administering medication. Assess the site on the patient where the injection is to be given. Avoid sites that are bruised, tender, hard, swollen, inflamed, or scarred. These conditions could affect absorption (ADA, 2015; Gelder, 2014). Assess the patient's knowledge of the medication. If the patient has deficient knowledge about the medication, this may be the appropriate time to begin education about it. If the medication may affect the patient's vital signs, assess them before administration. If the medication is for pain relief, assess the patient's pain before and after administration. Verify patient name, dose, route, and time of administration.

NURSING DIAGNOSIS	Determine related factors for the nursing diagnoses based on the patient's current status. Appropriate nursing diagnoses may include: • Deficient knowledge • Risk for infection • Risk for injury

OUTCOME IDENTIFICATION AND PLANNING	The expected outcome to achieve is that the patient receives the medication via the subcutaneous route and experiences the intended effect of the medication. Other outcomes that may be appropriate include the following: the patient does not experience adverse effects; and the patient understands and complies with the medication regimen.

IMPLEMENTATION

ACTION	RATIONALE
1. Gather equipment. Check each medication order against the original order in the medical record, according to facility policy. Clarify any inconsistencies. Check the patient's health record for allergies.	This comparison helps to identify errors that may have occurred when orders were transcribed. The primary care provider's order or prescription is the legal record of medication orders for each facility.
2. Know the actions, special nursing considerations, safe dose ranges, purpose of administration, and adverse effects of the medications to be administered. Consider the appropriateness of the medication for this patient.	This knowledge aids the nurse in evaluating the therapeutic effect of the medication in relation to the patient's disorder and can also be used to educate the patient about the medication.
3. Perform hand hygiene.	Hand hygiene prevents the spread of microorganisms.

(continued)

Skill 7 ▶ Administering a Subcutaneous Injection *(continued)*

ACTION	RATIONALE
4. Move the medication supply system to the outside of the patient's room or prepare for administration at the medication supply system in the medication area. Alternatively, access the medication administration supply system at or inside the patient's room.	Organization facilitates error-free administration and saves time.
5. Unlock the medication supply system or drawer. Enter pass code and scan employee identification, if required.	Locking the medication supply system or drawer safeguards each patient's medication supply. Facility accrediting organizations require medication supply systems to be locked when not in use. Entering pass code and scanning ID allows only authorized users into the computer system and identifies the user for documentation by the computer.
6. Prepare medications for one patient at a time.	This prevents errors in medication administration.
7. Read the eMAR/MAR and select the proper medication from the medication supply system or the patient's medication drawer.	This is the *first* check of the label.
8. Compare the medication label with the eMAR/MAR. Check expiration dates and perform calculations, if necessary. Scan the bar code on the package, if required.	This is the *second* check of the label. Verify calculations with another nurse to ensure safety, if necessary.
9. If necessary, withdraw medication from an ampule or vial as described in Skills 3 and 4.	
10. Depending on facility policy, the third check of the label may occur at this point. If so, when all medications for one patient have been prepared, recheck the labels with the eMAR/MAR before taking the medications to the patient. However, many facilities require the third check to occur at the bedside, after identifying the patient.	This *third* check ensures accuracy and helps to prevent errors. *Note:* Many facilities require the *third* check to occur at the bedside, after identifying the patient and before administration.
11. Lock the medication supply system before leaving it.	Locking the medication supply system or drawer safeguards the patient's medication supply. Facility accrediting organizations require medication supply systems to be locked when not in use.
12. Transport medications to the patient's bedside carefully, and keep the medications in sight at all times.	Careful handling and close observation prevent accidental or deliberate disarrangement of medications.
13. Ensure that the patient receives the medications at the correct time.	Check facility policy, which may allow for administration within a period of 30 minutes before or 30 minutes after the designated time.
14. Perform hand hygiene and put on PPE, if indicated.	Hand hygiene and PPE prevent the spread of microorganisms. PPE is required based on transmission precautions.
15. Identify the patient. Compare the information with the eMAR/MAR. The patient should be identified using at least two of the following methods (The Joint Commission, 2018):	Identifying the patient ensures the right patient receives the medications and helps prevent errors. The patient's room number or physical location is not used as an identifier (The Joint Commission, 2018). Replace the identification band if it is missing or inaccurate in any way.
a. Check the name on the patient's identification band.	
b. Check the identification number on the patient's identification band.	
c. Check the birth date on the patient's identification band.	
d. Ask the patient to state his or her name and birth date, based on facility policy.	This requires a response from the patient, but illness and strange surroundings often cause patients to be confused.

ACTION	RATIONALE
16. Close the door to the room or pull the bedside curtain.	This provides patient privacy.
17. **Complete necessary assessments before administering medications. Check the patient's allergy bracelet or ask the patient about allergies. Explain the purpose and action of the medication to the patient.**	Assessment is a prerequisite to administration of medications. Explanation provides rationale, increases knowledge, and reduces anxiety.
18. Scan the patient's bar code on the identification band, if required (Figure 2).	Scanning provides an additional check to ensure that the medication is given to the right patient.

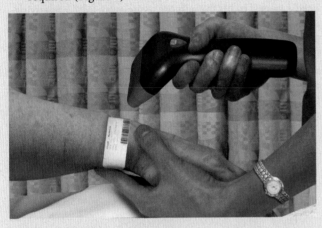

FIGURE 2. Scanning bar code on the patient's identification bracelet. (*Photo by B. Proud.*)

ACTION	RATIONALE
19. **Based on facility policy, the third check of the label may occur at this point. If so, recheck the labels with the eMAR/MAR before administering the medications to the patient.**	Many facilities require the *third* check to occur at the bedside, after identifying the patient and before administration. If facility policy directs the *third* check at this time, this *third* check ensures accuracy and helps to prevent errors.
20. Put on clean gloves.	Gloves help prevent exposure to contaminants.
21. Select an appropriate administration site.	Appropriate site prevents injury and allows for accurate reading of the test site at the appropriate time.
22. Assist the patient to the appropriate position for the site chosen. Drape, as needed, to expose only site area to be used.	Appropriate site prevents injury. Draping helps maintain the patient's privacy.
23. Identify the appropriate landmarks for the site chosen.	Good visualization is necessary to establish the correct site location and to avoid tissue damage.
24. Cleanse the area around the injection site with an antimicrobial swab. Use a firm, circular motion while moving outward from the injection site (Figure 3). Allow the area to dry.	Pathogens on the skin can be forced into the tissues by the needle. Moving from the center outward prevents contamination of the site. Allowing the antimicrobial solution to dry completely (15 to 30 seconds) ensures complete antimicrobial effectiveness (Harper, 2014), and prevents introducing alcohol into the tissue, which can be irritating and uncomfortable.

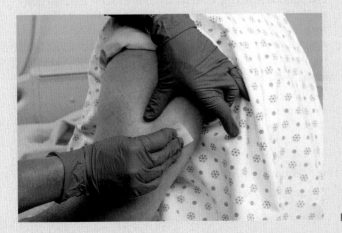

FIGURE 3. Cleaning injection site.

(continued)

Skill 7 ▶ Administering a Subcutaneous Injection *(continued)*

ACTION	RATIONALE
25. Remove the needle cap with the nondominant hand, pulling it straight off.	The cap protects the needle from contact with microorganisms. This technique lessens the risk of an accidental needlestick.
26. Create a skin fold, if necessary, by pinching the area surrounding the injection site. Alternatively, spread the skin taut at the site, based on assessment of the patient and needle length used for the injection (Figure 4).	Decision to create a skin fold is based on the nurse's assessment of the patient and needle length used. Recommendations differ regarding pinching a skin fold for administration. Pinching is advised for thinner patients and when a longer needle is used to lift the adipose tissue away from underlying muscle and tissue (Gelder, 2014; Sexson et al., 2016). If skin is pulled taut, it may provide less painful entry into the subcutaneous tissue.
27. Hold the syringe in the dominant hand between the thumb and forefinger. Inject the needle quickly at a 45- or 90-degree angle, depending on the amount of underlying subcutaneous tissue. (Figure 5).	Inserting the needle quickly causes less pain to the patient. For a person with a limited amount of subcutaneous tissue, insert the needle at a 45-degree angle.

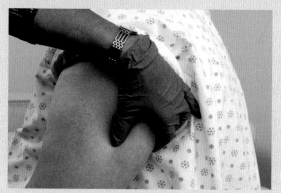

FIGURE 4. Pinching the area surrounding the injection site to create a skin fold, if necessary.

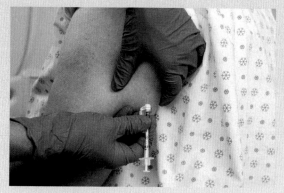

FIGURE 5. Inserting needle.

28. If pinching is used, once the needle is inserted, release the skin and stabilize the base of the needle to avoid injecting into the compressed tissue. Slide your dominant hand to the end of the plunger. Avoid moving the syringe.	Injecting the solution into compressed tissues results in pressure against nerve fibers and creates discomfort. Stabilizing the base of the needle secures the syringe. Moving the syringe could cause damage to the tissues and inadvertent administration into an incorrect area.
29. Inject the medication slowly (at a rate of 10 sec/mL).	Rapid injection of the solution creates pressure in the tissues, resulting in discomfort.
30. Withdraw the needle quickly at the same angle at which it was inserted, while supporting the surrounding tissue with your nondominant hand.	Slow withdrawal of the needle pulls the tissues and causes discomfort. Applying counter traction around the injection site helps to prevent pulling on the tissue as the needle is withdrawn. Removing the needle at the same angle at which it was inserted minimizes tissue damage and discomfort for the patient.
31. Do not recap the used needle. Engage the safety shield or needle guard.	Safety shield or needle guard prevents accidental needlestick.
32. If blood or clear fluid appears at the site after withdrawing the needle, use a gauze square to apply gentle pressure to the site. **Do not massage the site.**	Massaging the site can damage underlying tissue and increase the absorption of the medication. Massaging after heparin administration can contribute to hematoma formation.
33. Assist the patient to a position of comfort.	This provides for the well-being of the patient.

ACTION	RATIONALE
34. Discard the needle and syringe in the appropriate receptacle.	Proper disposal of the needle prevents injury.
35. Remove gloves and additional PPE, if used. Perform hand hygiene.	Proper removal of PPE reduces the risk for infection transmission and contamination of other items. Hand hygiene prevents the spread of microorganisms.
36. Document the administration of the medication immediately after administration.	Timely documentation helps to ensure patient safety.
37. Evaluate the patient's response to the medication within the appropriate time frame for the particular medication.	The patient needs to be evaluated for therapeutic and adverse effects from the medication.

EVALUATION

The expected outcomes have been met when the patient receives the medication via the subcutaneous route and experiences the intended effect of the medication; the patient does not experience adverse effects; and the patient understands and complies with the medication regimen.

DOCUMENTATION

Guidelines

Record each medication given on the eMAR/MAR or health record using the required format immediately after administration, including date, dose, time, and the site of administration. If using a bar-code system, medication administration is automatically recorded when the bar code is scanned. PRN medications require documentation of the reason for administration. Prompt recording avoids the possibility of accidentally repeating the administration of the drug. If the drug was refused or omitted, record this in the appropriate area on the medication record and notify the primary care provider. This verifies the reason medication was omitted and ensures that health care personnel providing care for the patient are aware of the occurrence.

UNEXPECTED SITUATIONS AND ASSOCIATED INTERVENTIONS

- *When skin fold is released, needle pulls out of skin:* Engage safety shield or needle guard. Appropriately discard needle. Attach new needle to syringe and administer injection.
- *Patient refuses to let you administer medication in a different location:* Explain the rationale behind rotating injection sites. Discuss other available injection sites with the patient. If the patient will still not allow injection in another area, administer medication to patient, document patient's refusal of rotation of injection site and discussion, and notify primary care provider.
- *You stick yourself with the needle before injection:* Discard needle and syringe appropriately. Follow facility policy regarding needlestick injury. Prepare new syringe with medication and administer to patient. Complete appropriate paperwork and follow facility's policy regarding accidental needlestick injuries.
- *You stick yourself with the needle after injection:* Discard needle and syringe appropriately. Complete appropriate paperwork and follow facility's policy regarding accidental needlestick injuries.
- *During injection, patient pulls away from the needle before the medication is delivered fully:* Remove and appropriately discard needle. Attach a new needle to syringe and administer remaining medication at a different site. Document events and interventions according to facility policy.

SPECIAL CONSIDERATIONS

General Considerations

- Ongoing assessment is an important part of nursing care for both evaluation of patient response to administered medications and early detection of adverse drug reactions. If an adverse effect is suspected, withhold further medication doses and notify the patient's primary care provider. Additional intervention is based on type of reaction and patient assessment.

(continued)

Skill 7 ▶ Administering a Subcutaneous Injection *(continued)*

- Because absorption rates vary from site to site, it is recommended that patients administering their own insulin use the same area of the body at the same time every day to ensure more consistent absorption and prevent tissue changes from repeated use of the same site (Frandsen & Pennington, 2014; ADA, 2015). For instance, every morning the patient may use the abdomen for insulin injection, and every evening before dinner, the patient may inject the insulin into the arms or thighs. Keep in mind that the best absorption occurs in the abdomen. In each case, the injections should be given an inch away from the previous injection site so that the same area will not be used again in the same month. A small spot bandage or piece of tape can be used to mark the first injection site, with subsequent injections rotated in a circle around that site. After this area has been used, an adjacent site, an inch away, can be selected, using the same rotation format. A marked diagram incorporated into the patient's plan of care is also helpful for noting alternative sites. Do not rely on memory. The patient cannot always recall the site of the previous injection, thus the site of administration should be recorded; when the patient is receiving care from a health care provider, the site of administration must be recorded in the patient's health record.
- Heparin is administered subcutaneously. The abdomen is the most commonly used administration site. Avoid the area 2 in around the umbilicus and the belt line.
- Certain medications have specific manufacturer-recommended administration requirements. For example, enoxaparin (low–molecular-weight heparin) should be administered alternating between the left and right anterolateral and left and right posterolateral abdominal wall ("love handles") (Sanofi Aventis, 2013, 2016) (Figure 6). To administer the medication, pinch the tissue gently to form a skin fold and insert the needle at a 90-degree angle (Sanofi Aventis, 2016). In addition, enoxaparin is packaged in a prefilled syringe with an air bubble. Do not expel the air bubble before administration.

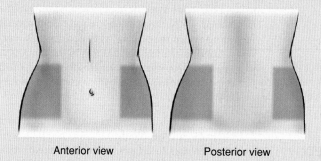

Anterior view   Posterior view

FIGURE 6. Sites for administration of enoxaparin.

Infant and Child Considerations
- Do not tell a child that an injection will not hurt. Describe the feel of the injection as a pinch or a sting. A child who believes you have been dishonest with him/her is less likely to cooperate with future procedures.

Older Adult Considerations
- Many older adults have less adipose tissue. Adjust the needle length and insertion angle accordingly. (Refer to discussion earlier in Skill.) You do not want to inadvertently give a subcutaneous medication intramuscularly.

Home Care Considerations
- Reuse of syringes in the home setting is not recommended.
- The use of antimicrobial swabs to clean the injection site in home environments may be unnecessary; patients may use soap and water to clean the site if the area is visibly soiled (Sexson et al., 2016).
- Because absorption rates vary from site to site, it is recommended that patients administering their own insulin use the same area of the body at the same time every day to ensure more consistent absorption and prevent tissue changes from repeated use of the same site (Frandsen & Pennington, 2014; ADA, 2015). Refer to the information discussed in the "General Considerations" section of this Skill.
- Encourage patients to consult the policies of their local government regarding contaminated and sharps waste disposal. Depending on local requirements, patients may dispose of needles and syringes in a hard, plastic container. Liquid detergent or liquid fabric softener containers are good choices. Never use glass containers.

Skill Variation ▶ Using an Insulin Injection Pen to Administer Insulin via the Subcutaneous Route

Prepare medication as outlined in steps 1–23 above (Skill 7).

1. Remove the pen cap.
2. Insert an insulin cartridge into the pen, if necessary, following the manufacturer's directions.
3. If administering an insulin suspension, gently roll the pen 10 times and invert the pen 10 times to mix the insulin.
4. Scrub the self-sealing seal end of the pen cartridge holder with an antimicrobial swab.
5. Remove the protective paper tab from the needle.
6. Screw the needle onto the reservoir.
7. Remove the outer and inner needle caps. (Patients at home should reserve the outer shield for later use.)
8. Dial the dose selector to 2 units to prime the pen (perform an "air shot") to get rid of air and make certain the pen is working properly.
9. Hold the pen upright and tap to force any air bubbles to the top.
10. Hold the pen upright and press the injection button or plunger firmly. Watch for a drop of insulin at the needle tip.
11. Check the drug reservoir to make sure sufficient insulin is available for the dose.
12. Check that the dose selector is at "0," then dial the units of insulin for the dose.
13. Put on gloves.
14. Clean the injection site. If the pen needle is longer than 5 mm, gently pinch the skin at the injection site to form a skin fold (Becton, Dickinson and Company, 2016a).
15. Hold the pen in the palm of the hand, perpendicular to the forearm, with the thumb at the injection button end of the pen. Use the thumb for injection (Figure A).
16. Administer the subcutaneous injection. Press the injection button on the pen all the way in. Keep the button depressed and count to 10 before removing from the skin.
17. The safety shield automatically covers the needle when needle is removed from the skin. Remove the needle

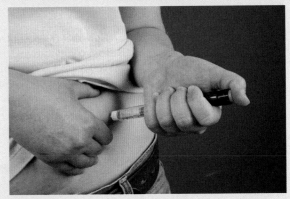

FIGURE A. Patient using insulin pen. (*Photo by B. Proud.*)

from the pen; a second safety shield automatically covers the back end of the needle when removed from the pen. Dispose of the needle in a sharps container.

18. Alternatively, patients at home should replace the reserved outer shield on the needle before removing the needle from the pen. Other needle removal devices and procedures exist; patients should follow the instructions provided by their health care provider related to their specific insulin pen.
19. Remove gloves and additional PPE, if used.

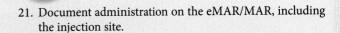 20. Perform hand hygiene.

21. Document administration on the eMAR/MAR, including the injection site.

Source: Adapted from Becton, Dickinson and Company. (2016a). How to inject with a pen. Retrieved https://www.bd.com/en-us/company/video-gallery?video=4592430149001; Becton, Dickinson and Company. (2016b). Safety needles. Retrieved http://www.bd.com/hypodermic/products/autoshield/duo

Skill 8 ▶ Administering an Intramuscular Injection

Intramuscular injections deliver medication through the skin and subcutaneous tissues into certain muscles. Muscles have a larger and a greater number of blood vessels than subcutaneous tissue, allowing faster onset of action than with subcutaneous injections. An intramuscular injection is chosen when a reasonably rapid systemic uptake of the drug is needed by the body and when a relatively prolonged action is required. Some medications administered intramuscularly are formulated to have a longer duration of effect. The deposit of medication creates a depot at the injection site, designed to deliver slow, sustained release over hours, days, or weeks.

(continued)

It is important to choose the right needle length for a particular intramuscular injection. Needle length should be based on the individual patient. (See Table 8-1 for intramuscular needle length recommendations.) Patients who are obese may require a longer needle, and emaciated patients may require a shorter needle. Appropriate gauge is determined by the medication being administered. In general, biologic agents and medications in aqueous solutions should be administered with a 20- to 25-gauge needle. Medications in oil-based solutions should be administered with an 18- to 25-gauge needle. Many medications come in prefilled syringe units. If a needle is provided on the prefilled unit, ensure that the needle on the unit is the appropriate length for the patient and situation.

To avoid complications, the nurse must be able to identify anatomic landmarks and site boundaries. See Figure 1 for a depiction of anatomic landmarks and site boundaries for potential intramuscular injection sites. Consider the age of the patient, medication type, and medication volume when selecting an intramuscular injection site. (See Table 8-2 for information related to intramuscular site selection.) Rotate the sites used to administer intramuscular medications when therapy requires repeated injections. Depending on the site selected, it may be necessary to reposition the patient (refer to Table 8-3).

Table 8-1 | Intramuscular Injection Needle Length

SITE/AGE	NEEDLE LENGTH
Vastus lateralis	5⁄8″ to 1¼″
Deltoid (children)	5⁄8″ to 1¼″
Deltoid (adults)	1″ to 1½″
Ventrogluteal (adults)	1½″

Note: Biological sex and weight are directly related to needle length choice; the size of the muscle, the adipose tissue thickness at the injection site, the volume of medication to be administered, and the injection technique also need to be considered.

Source: Adapted from Centers for Disease Control and Prevention (CDC). (2015a). Chapter 6. Vaccine administration. *The pink book.* Retrieved https://www.cdc.gov/vaccines/pubs/pinkbook/vac-admin.html; Centers for Disease Control and Prevention (CDC). (2015b). In J. Hamborsky, A. Kroger, & S. Wolfe (Eds.). *Epidemiology and prevention of vaccine-preventable diseases* (13th ed.). Washington, DC: Public Health Foundation. Retrieved http://www.cdc.gov/vaccines/pubs/pinkbook/index.html; and *Nicoll, L., & Hesby, A.* (2002). Intramuscular injection: An integrative research review and guideline for evidence-based practice. *Applied Nursing Research, 16*(2), 149–162.

Table 8-2 | Intramuscular Site Selection

AGE OF PATIENT	RECOMMENDED SITE
Infants	Vastus lateralis
Toddlers (1–2 years)	Vastus lateralis (preferred) or deltoid
Child/Adolescent (3–18 years)	Deltoid (preferred) or vastus lateralis
Adults	Deltoid (vaccines) or ventrogluteal (general IM injections)

Source: Adapted from Centers for Disease Control and Prevention (CDC). (2015a). Chapter 6. Vaccine administration. *The pink book.* Retrieved https://www.cdc.gov/vaccines/pubs/pinkbook/vac-admin.html; and Nicoll, L., & Hesby, A. (2002). Intramuscular injection: An integrative research review and guideline for evidence-based practice. *Applied Nursing Research, 16*(2), 149–162.

Table 8-3 | Patient Positioning

INJECTION SITE	PATIENT POSITION
Deltoid	Patient may sit or stand. A child may be held in an adult's lap.
Ventrogluteal	Patient may stand, sit, lie laterally, and lie supine.
Vastus lateralis	Patient may sit or lie supine. Infants and young children may lie supine or be held in an adult's lap.

Source: Adapted from Centers for Disease Control and Prevention (CDC). (2015a). Chapter 6. Vaccine administration. *The pink book.* Retrieved https://www.cdc.gov/vaccines/pubs/pinkbook/vac-admin.html.

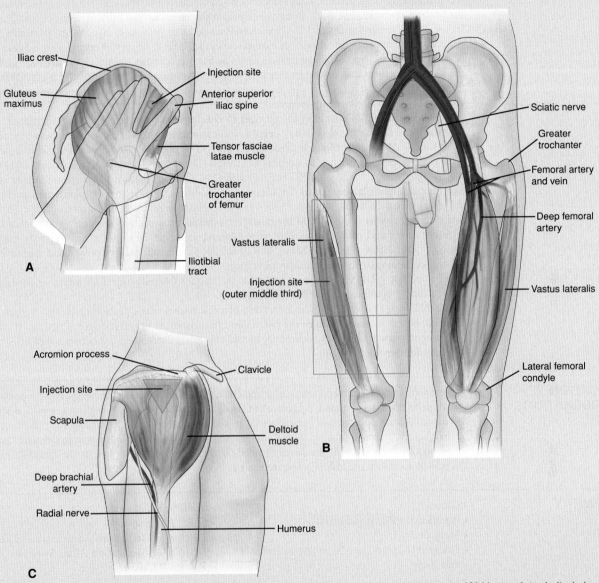

FIGURE 1. Sites for intramuscular injections. Descriptions for locating sites are given in the text. (**A**) Ventrogluteal site is located by placing palm on greater trochanter and index finger toward the anterosuperior iliac spine. (**B**) Vastus lateralis site is identified by dividing the thigh into thirds, horizontally and vertically. (**C**) Deltoid muscle site is located by palpating lower edge of acromion process.

Administer the intramuscular injection so that the needle is perpendicular to the patient's body. This ensures it is given using an injection angle between 72 and 90 degrees, with the goal of 90 degrees (CDC, 2015b; Katsma & Katsma, 2000). The angle of insertion for intramuscular injections.

The medication volume that can be administered intramuscularly varies based on the intended site. In general, 1 to 5 mL is the accepted volume range, with a limitation of 1 mL of solution at the deltoid site. However, up to 2 mL may be administered at the deltoid site, depending on the size of the muscle (Hunt, 2008). The less-developed muscles of children and older people limit the intramuscular injection to 1 to 2 mL.

Many of the drugs given intramuscularly can cause irritation to subcutaneous tissues when backflow into the tissues occurs along the injection track. Therefore, the Z-track technique is

(continued)

Skill 8 ▶ Administering an Intramuscular Injection *(continued)*

recommended for all intramuscular injections (particularly nonvaccine injections) to ensure that medication does not leak back along the needle track and into the subcutaneous tissue (Nicoll & Hesby, 2002; Zimmerman, 2010). This technique reduces pain and discomfort, particularly for patients receiving injections over an extended period. The Z-track method is also suggested for older adults who have decreased muscle mass. Some medications, such as iron, are best given via the Z-track method due to the irritation and discoloration associated with the medication. The decision regarding stretching or pinching the skin, or using the Z-track method is based on the individual patient and nursing judgment.

Aspiration, or pulling back on the plunger to check that a blood vessel has been entered, is not necessary and has not proved to be a reliable indicator of needle placement. Despite a tradition of aspiration, if correct technique is used, the likelihood of injecting into a blood vessel is small and there is no scientific evidence to support aspiration (Davidson & Rourke, 2013; Sisson, 2015). The World Health Organization (WHO) (2016) and CDC (2015b) continue to recommend no aspiration for intramuscular injections. In addition, aspiration causes increased pain when performed over the standard 5 to 10 seconds (Sisson). Some literature suggests that aspiration may be indicated when administering certain medications (nonvaccines, such as the antibiotic penicillin), at certain dosages and certain rates, but more research needs to be done on this topic in the adult setting (CDC, 2015b; Thomas, Mraz, & Rajcan, 2015). Consult facility policy and manufacturer recommendations to ensure safe administration.

Refer to Box 7-1 in Skill 7 on page 34 for techniques for reducing discomfort when injecting medications subcutaneously or intramuscularly.

The following skill outlines administration of an intramuscular injection using the Z-track technique. If, based on assessment of the particular circumstances for an individual patient, the nurse decides not to use the Z-track technique, the skin should be stretched flat between two fingers and held taut for needle insertion.

DELEGATION CONSIDERATIONS

The administration of an intramuscular injection is not delegated to nursing assistive personnel (NAP) or to unlicensed assistive personnel (UAP). Depending on the state's nurse practice act and the organization's policies and procedures, the administration of an intramuscular injection may be delegated to licensed practical/vocational nurses (LPN/LVNs). The decision to delegate must be based on careful analysis of the patient's needs and circumstances, as well as the qualifications of the person to whom the task is being delegated.

EQUIPMENT

- Gloves
- Additional PPE, as indicated
- Medication
- Sterile syringe and needle of appropriate size and gauge

- Antimicrobial swab
- Small gauze square
- Electronic Medication Administration Record (eMAR) or Medication Administration Record (MAR)

ASSESSMENT

Assess the appropriateness of the drug for the patient. Review medical history, allergy, assessment, and laboratory data that may influence drug administration. Check the expiration date before administering the medication. Assess the site on the patient where the injection is to be given. Avoid any site that is bruised, tender, hard, swollen, inflamed, or scarred. Assess the patient's knowledge of the medication. If the patient has deficient knowledge about the medication, this may be the appropriate time to begin education about it. If the medication may affect the patient's vital signs, assess them before administration. If the medication is intended for pain relief, assess the patient's pain before and after administration. Verify patient name, dose, route, and time of administration.

NURSING DIAGNOSIS

Determine related factors for the nursing diagnoses based on the patient's current status. Appropriate diagnoses may include:

- Deficient knowledge
- Risk for injury
- Risk for infection

OUTCOME IDENTIFICATION AND PLANNING

The expected outcome to achieve when administering an intramuscular injection is that the patient receives the medication via the intramuscular route and experiences the intended effect of the medication; the patient does not experience adverse effects; and the patient understands and complies with the medication regimen.

IMPLEMENTATION

ACTION	RATIONALE
1. Gather equipment. Check each medication order against the original order in the health record according to facility policy. Clarify any inconsistencies. Check the patient's health record for allergies.	This comparison helps to identify errors that may have occurred when orders were transcribed. The primary care provider's order or prescription is the legal record of medication orders for each facility.
2. Know the actions, special nursing considerations, safe dose ranges, purpose of administration, and adverse effects of the medications to be administered. Consider the appropriateness of the medication for this patient.	This knowledge aids the nurse in evaluating the therapeutic effect of the medication in relation to the patient's disorder and can also be used to educate the patient about the medication.
3. Perform hand hygiene.	Hand hygiene prevents the spread of microorganisms.
4. Move the medication supply system to the outside of the patient's room or prepare for administration at the medication supply system in the medication area. Alternatively, access the medication administration supply system at or inside the patient's room.	Organization facilitates error-free administration and saves time.
5. Unlock the medication supply system or drawer. Enter pass code and scan employee identification, if required.	Locking the medication supply system or drawer safeguards each patient's medication supply. Facility accrediting organizations require medication supply systems to be locked when not in use. Entering pass code and scanning ID allows only authorized users into the system and identifies the user for documentation by the computer.
6. **Prepare medications for one patient at a time.**	This prevents errors in medication administration.
7. Read the eMAR/MAR and select the proper medication from medication supply system or the patient's medication drawer.	This is the *first* check of the label.
8. Compare the label with the eMAR/MAR. Check expiration dates and perform calculations, if necessary. Scan the bar code on the package, if required.	This is the *second* check of the label. Verify calculations with another nurse to ensure safety, if necessary.
9. If necessary, withdraw medication from an ampule or vial as described in Skills 3 and 4.	
10. **Depending on facility policy, the third check of the label may occur at this point. If so, when all medications for one patient have been prepared, recheck the labels with the eMAR/MAR before taking the medications to the patient. However, many facilities require the third check to occur at the bedside, after identifying the patient.**	This *third* check ensures accuracy and helps to prevent errors. *Note:* Many facilities require the *third* check to occur at the bedside, after identifying the patient and before administration.
11. **Lock the medication supply system before leaving it.**	Locking the medication supply system or drawer safeguards the patient's medication supply. Facility accrediting organizations require medication supply systems to be locked when not in use.
12. Transport medications to the patient's bedside carefully, and keep the medications in sight at all times.	Careful handling and close observation prevent accidental or deliberate disarrangement of medications.

(continued)

Skill 8 ▶ Administering an Intramuscular Injection *(continued)*

ACTION	RATIONALE

13. Ensure that the patient receives the medications at the correct time.

Check facility policy, which may allow for administration within a period of 30 minutes before or 30 minutes after the designated time.

14. Perform hand hygiene and put on PPE, if indicated.

Hand hygiene and PPE prevent the spread of microorganisms. PPE is required based on transmission precautions.

15. Identify the patient. Compare the information with the eMAR/MAR. The patient should be identified using at least two of the following methods (The Joint Commission, 2018):

Identifying the patient ensures the right patient receives the medications and helps prevent errors. The patient's room number or physical location is not used as an identifier (The Joint Commission, 2018). Replace the identification band if it is missing or inaccurate in any way.

   a. Check the name on the patient's identification band.

   b. Check the identification number on the patient's identification band.

   c. Check the birth date on the patient's identification band.

   d. Ask the patient to state his or her name and birth date, based on facility policy.

This requires a response from the patient, but illness and strange surroundings often cause patients to be confused.

16. Close the door to the room or pull the bedside curtain.

This provides patient privacy.

17. Complete necessary assessments before administering medications. Check the patient's allergy bracelet or ask the patient about allergies. Explain the purpose and action of the medication to the patient.

Assessment is a prerequisite to administration of medications. Explanation provides rationale, increases knowledge, and reduces anxiety.

18. Scan the patient's bar code on the identification band, if required (Figure 2).

Provides an additional check to ensure that the medication is given to the right patient.

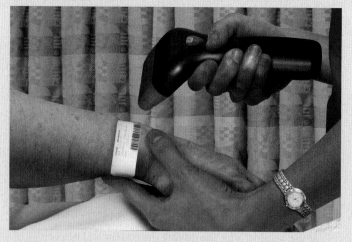

FIGURE 2. Scanning bar code on the patient's identification bracelet. (*Photo by B. Proud.*)

19. Based on facility policy, the third check of the label may occur at this point. If so, recheck the labels with the eMAR/MAR before administering the medications to the patient.

Many facilities require the *third* check to occur at the bedside, after identifying the patient and before administration. If facility policy directs the *third* check at this time, this *third* check ensures accuracy and helps to prevent errors.

20. Put on clean gloves.

Gloves help prevent exposure to contaminants.

21. Select an appropriate administration site.

Selecting the appropriate site prevents injury.

22. Assist the patient to the appropriate position for the site chosen. See Table 8-3. Drape, as needed, to expose only the site area being used.

Appropriate positioning for the site chosen prevents injury. Draping helps maintain the patient's privacy.

ACTION	RATIONALE

23. Identify the appropriate landmarks for the site chosen (Figure 3).

Good visualization is necessary to establish the correct site location and to avoid tissue damage.

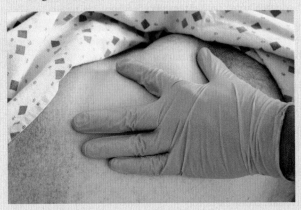

FIGURE 3. Identifying the appropriate landmarks.

24. Cleanse the area around the injection site with an antimicrobial swab. Use a firm, circular motion while moving outward from the injection site. Allow the area to dry.

Pathogens on the skin can be forced into the tissues by the needle. Moving from the center outward prevents contamination of the site. Allowing the antimicrobial solution to dry completely (15 to 30 seconds) ensures complete antimicrobial effectiveness (Harper, 2014), and prevents introducing alcohol into the tissue, which can be irritating and uncomfortable.

25. Remove the needle cap by pulling it straight off. Hold the syringe in your dominant hand between the thumb and forefinger.

This technique lessens the risk of an accidental needlestick and also prevents inadvertently unscrewing the needle from the barrel of the syringe.

26. Displace the skin in a Z-track manner. Pull the skin and underlying tissue down or to one side about 1 in (2.5 cm) with your nondominant hand and hold the skin and tissue in this position (Figure 4). Hand and fingers should remain in the appropriate position for the site chosen to continue accurate identification of landmarks and ensure safe injection technique. Alternatively, if, based on assessment of the particular circumstances for an individual patient, the nurse decides not to use the Z-Track technique, the skin should be stretched flat between two fingers and held taut for needle insertion.

Z-track technique is recommended for all intramuscular injections to ensure medication does not leak back along the needle track and into the subcutaneous tissue (Nicoll & Hesby, 2002; Zimmerman, 2010). This technique reduces pain and discomfort, particularly for patients receiving injections over an extended period. The Z-track method is also suggested for older adults who have decreased muscle mass. Some agents, such as iron, are best given via the Z-track method due to the irritation and discoloration associated with this agent.

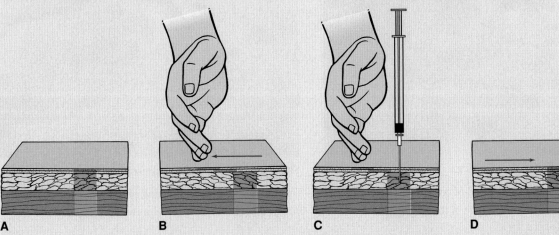

FIGURE 4. Z-track or zigzag technique is recommended for intramuscular injections. (**A**) Normal skin and tissues. (**B**) Moving skin to one side. (**C**) Needle is inserted at a 90-degree angle. (**D**) Once needle is withdrawn, displaced tissue is allowed to return to its normal position, preventing solution from escaping from muscle tissue. Hand and finger positioning is adjusted for the specific administration site for accurate identification of landmarks and use of safe injection technique.

(continued)

Skill 8 ▶ Administering an Intramuscular Injection *(continued)*

27. Quickly dart the needle into the tissue so that the needle is perpendicular to the patient's body, with the goal of an angle of 90 degrees (Figure 5).

28. As soon as the needle is in place, use the thumb and forefinger of your nondominant hand to hold the lower end of the syringe, taking care to maintain the displacement of the skin and tissue. Slide your dominant hand to the end of the plunger. Inject the solution slowly (10 sec/mL of medication).

29. Once the medication has been instilled, wait 10 seconds before withdrawing the needle.

30. Withdraw the needle smoothly and steadily at the same angle at which it was inserted, supporting tissue around the injection site with your nondominant hand. **Remove the hand holding the displaced skin and tissue only after removal of the needle.**

31. Do not recap the used needle. Engage the safety shield or needle guard, if present.

32. Apply gentle pressure at the site with a dry gauze (Figure 6). **Do not massage the site.**

A quick injection is less painful. Inserting the needle at a 90-degree angle is the goal; actual administration using a 72- to 90-degree angle facilitates entry into muscle tissue.

Moving the syringe could cause damage to the tissues and inadvertent administration into an incorrect area. Rapid injection of the solution creates pressure in the tissues, resulting in discomfort. Aspiration, or pulling back on the plunger to check that a blood vessel has been entered, is not necessary and has not proved to be a reliable indicator of needle placement (Davidson & Rourke, 2013; Sisson, 2015). Some literature suggests that aspiration may be indicated when administering certain medications, at certain dosages, at certain rates, but more research needs to be done on this topic in the adult setting (CDC, 2015b; Thomas, Mraz, & Rajcan, 2015). Consult facility policy and manufacturer recommendations to ensure safe administration.

Allows medication to begin to diffuse into the surrounding muscle tissue (Nicoll & Hesby, 2002).

Slow withdrawal of the needle pulls the tissues and causes discomfort. Applying counter traction around the injection site helps to prevent pulling on the tissue as the needle is withdrawn. Removing the needle at the same angle at which it was inserted minimizes tissue damage and discomfort for the patient. Allowing displaced skin and tissue to move back into place while needle is still inserted causes damage to the tissues

Safety shield or needle guard prevents accidental needlestick.

Light pressure causes less trauma and irritation to the tissues. Massaging can force medication into subcutaneous tissues and increase discomfort.

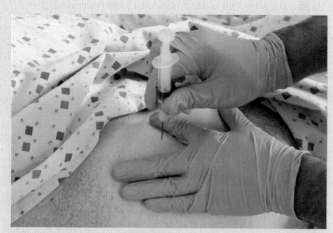

FIGURE 5. Darting needle into tissue.

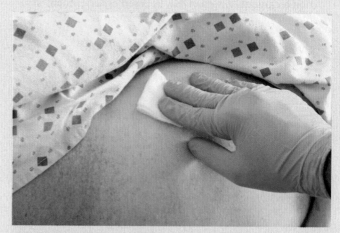

FIGURE 6. Applying gentle pressure at injection site.

33. Assist the patient to a position of comfort.

34. Discard the needle and syringe in the appropriate receptacle.

This provides for the well-being of the patient.

Proper disposal of the needle prevents injury.

ACTION	RATIONALE
35. Remove gloves and additional PPE, if used. Perform hand hygiene.	Proper removal of PPE reduces the risk for infection transmission and contamination of other items. Hand hygiene prevents the spread of microorganisms.
36. Document the administration of the medication immediately after administration. See Documentation section below.	Timely documentation helps to ensure patient safety.
37. Evaluate the patient's response to the medication within the appropriate time frame. Assess site, if possible, within 2 to 4 hours after administration.	The patient needs to be evaluated for therapeutic and adverse effects from the medication. Visualization of the site allows for assessment of any untoward effects.

EVALUATION

The expected outcomes have been met when the patient receives the medication via the intramuscular route and experiences the intended effect of the medication; the patient does not experience adverse effects; and the patient understands and complies with the medication regimen.

DOCUMENTATION

Guidelines

Record each medication given on the eMAR/MAR or record using the required format, including date, time, and the site of administration, immediately after administration. If using a bar-code system, medication administration is automatically recorded when the bar code is scanned. PRN medications require documentation of the reason for administration. Prompt recording avoids the possibility of accidentally repeating the administration of the drug. If the drug was refused or omitted, record this in the appropriate area on the medication record and notify the primary care provider. This verifies the reason medication was omitted and ensures that health care personnel providing care for the patient are aware of the occurrence.

UNEXPECTED SITUATIONS AND ASSOCIATED INTERVENTIONS

- *You stick yourself with the needle before injection:* Discard needle and syringe appropriately. Follow facility policy regarding needlestick injury. Prepare new syringe with medication and administer to patient. Complete appropriate paperwork and follow facility's policy regarding accidental needlesticks.
- *You stick yourself with the needle after injection:* Discard needle and syringe appropriately. Follow facility policy regarding needlestick injury. Complete appropriate paperwork and follow facility's policy regarding accidental needlesticks.
- *During injection, the patient pulls away from the needle before the medication is delivered fully:* Remove and appropriately discard needle. Attach a new needle to syringe and administer remaining medication at a different site. Document events and interventions, according to facility policy.
- *While injecting the needle into the patient, you hit patient's bone:* Withdraw and discard the needle. Apply a new needle to the syringe and administer in an alternate site. Document incident in patient's medical record. Notify primary care provider. Complete appropriate paperwork related to special events, according to facility policy.

SPECIAL CONSIDERATIONS

General Considerations

- Ongoing assessment is an important part of nursing care for both evaluation of patient response to administered medications and early detection of adverse drug reactions. If an adverse effect is suspected, withhold further medication doses and notify the patient's primary care provider. Additional intervention is based on the type of reaction and patient assessment.
- The deltoid is the recommended site for vaccines for adults (CDC, 2015a).
- The ventrogluteal site is recommended for general IM injections in adults.

(continued)

Skill 8 ▶ Administering an Intramuscular Injection *(continued)*

Infant and Child Considerations

- The vastus lateralis is the preferred site for intramuscular injections in infants and young children (CDC, 2015a).
- The deltoid is the preferred site for children 3 through 18 years (CDC, 2015a).

Older Adult Considerations

- Muscle mass atrophies as a person ages. Take care to evaluate the patient's muscle mass and body composition. Use appropriate needle length and gauge for patient's body composition. Choose appropriate site based on the patient's body composition.

Home Care Considerations

- The use of antimicrobial swabs to clean the injection site in home environments may be unnecessary; patients may use soap and water to clean the site if the area is visibly soiled (Sexson et al., 2016).
- Encourage patients to consult the policies of their local government regarding contaminated and sharps waste disposal. Depending on local requirements, patients may dispose of needles and syringes in a hard, plastic container. Liquid detergent or liquid fabric softener containers are good choices. Never use glass containers.
- Reuse of syringes in the home setting is not recommended.

Skill 9 ▶ Administering a Continuous Subcutaneous Infusion: Applying an Insulin Pump

Some medications, such as insulin and morphine, may be administered continuously via the subcutaneous route. Continuous subcutaneous insulin infusion (CSII or insulin pump) allows for multiple preset rates of insulin delivery. This system uses a small, computerized reservoir that delivers insulin through infusion tubing to a small plastic cannula or needle or a wireless patch-pump system, that has no infusion set attached, inserted into the subcutaneous tissue (Phillips, 2016). The pump can be programmed to deliver multiple preset rates of insulin. The settings can be adjusted for exercise and illness, and bolus dose delivery can be timed in relation to meals. It is recommended that the site is changed every 2 to 3 days to prevent tissue damage or absorption problems (American Association of Diabetes Educators, 2014). Advantages of continuous subcutaneous medication infusion include the longer rate of absorption via the subcutaneous route and convenience for the patient. There are many different manufacturers of insulin pumps. Nurses need to be familiar with the particular pump in use by their patient and to refer to the specific manufacturer's recommendations for use. The following skill outlines steps in applying an insulin pump utilizing infusion tubing and a small needle-insertion device.

DELEGATION CONSIDERATIONS

The administration of a continuous subcutaneous infusion using an insulin pump is not delegated to nursing assistive personnel (NAP) or to unlicensed assistive personnel (UAP). Depending on the state's nurse practice act and the organization's policies and procedures, the management of an insulin pump in some settings may be delegated to licensed practical/vocational nurses (LPN/LVNs) who have received appropriate training. The decision to delegate must be based on careful analysis of the patient's needs and circumstances, as well as the qualifications of the person to whom the task is being delegated.

EQUIPMENT

- Insulin pump
- Pump syringe and vial of insulin or prefilled cartridge, as ordered
- Sterile infusion set
- Insertion (triggering) device
- Needle (24- or 22-gauge, or blunt-ended needle)

- Antimicrobial swabs
- Sterile nonocclusive dressing
- Electronic Medication Administration Record (eMAR) or Medication Administration Record (MAR)
- Disposable gloves
- Additional PPE, as indicated

ASSESSMENT	Assess the appropriateness of the drug for the patient. Review medical history, allergy, assessment, and laboratory data that may influence drug administration. Check the expiration date before administering the medication. Assess the infusion site. Typical infusion sites include those areas used for subcutaneous insulin injection. Assess the area where the pump is to be applied. Do not place the pump on skin that is irritated or not intact. Assess the patient's knowledge of the medication. If the patient has a knowledge deficit about the medication, this may be the appropriate time to begin education about it. Assess the patient's blood glucose level as appropriate or as ordered. Verify patient name, dose, route, and time of administration.

NURSING DIAGNOSIS	Determine related factors for the nursing diagnoses based on the patient's current status. Appropriate nursing diagnoses may include: • Deficient knowledge • Risk for unstable blood glucose level • Risk for infection

OUTCOME IDENTIFICATION AND PLANNING	The expected outcome is that the device is applied successfully, the medication is administered correctly, and the patient experiences the intended effect of the medication. Other outcomes that may be appropriate include the following: the patient understands the rationale for the pump use and mechanism of action; the patient's skin remains intact; pump is applied using aseptic technique; and the patient does not experience unstable blood glucose levels or adverse effect.

IMPLEMENTATION

ACTION	RATIONALE
1. Gather equipment. Check each medication order against the original order in the health record, according to facility policy. Clarify any inconsistencies. Check the patient's health record for allergies.	This comparison helps to identify errors that may have occurred when orders were transcribed. The primary care provider's order or prescription is the legal record of medication orders.
2. Know the actions, special nursing considerations, safe dose ranges, purpose of administration, and adverse effects of the medications to be administered. Consider the appropriateness of the medication for this patient.	This knowledge aids the nurse in evaluating the therapeutic effect of the medication in relation to the patient's disorder and can also be used to educate the patient about the medication.
3. Perform hand hygiene.	Hand hygiene prevents the spread of microorganisms.
4. Move the medication supply system to the outside of the patient's room or prepare for administration at the medication supply system in the medication area. Alternatively, access the medication administration supply system at or inside the patient's room.	Organization facilitates error-free administration and saves time.
5. Unlock the medication supply system or drawer. Enter pass code and scan employee identification, if required.	Locking the medication supply system or drawer safeguards each patient's medication supply. Facility accrediting organizations require medication supply systems to be locked when not in use. Entering pass code and scanning ID allows only authorized users into the system and identifies the user for documentation by the computer.
6. **Prepare medications for one patient at a time.**	This prevents errors in medication administration.
7. Read the eMAR/MAR and select the proper medication from medication supply system or the patient's medication drawer.	This is the *first* check of the label.

(*continued*)

Skill 9 ▶ Administering a Continuous Subcutaneous Infusion: Applying an Insulin Pump *(continued)*

ACTION	RATIONALE
8. Compare the label with the eMAR/MAR. Check expiration dates and perform calculations, if necessary. Scan the bar code on the package, if required.	This is the *second* check of the label. Verify calculations with another nurse to ensure safety, if necessary.
9. Attach a blunt-ended needle or a small-gauge needle to a syringe. Follow Skill 4 to prepare insulin from a vial, if necessary. Prepare enough insulin to last the patient 2 to 3 days, plus 30 units for priming tubing. If using a prepackaged insulin syringe or cartridge, remove from packaging.	Patient will wear pump for up to 3 days without changing syringe or tubing.
10. **Depending on facility policy, the third check of the label may occur at this point. If so, when all medications for one patient have been prepared, recheck the labels with the eMAR/MAR before taking the medications to the patient. However, many facilities require the third check to occur at the bedside, after identifying the patient.**	This *third* check ensures accuracy and helps to prevent errors. *Note:* Many facilities require the *third* check to occur at the bedside, after identifying the patient and before administration.
11. **Lock the medication supply system before leaving it.**	Locking the medication supply system or drawer safeguards the patient's medication supply. Facility accrediting organizations require medication supply systems to be locked when not in use.
12. **Transport medications to the patient's bedside carefully, and keep the medications in sight at all times.**	Careful handling and close observation prevent accidental or deliberate disarrangement of medications.
13. **Ensure that the patient receives the medications at the correct time.**	Check facility policy, which may allow for administration within a period of 30 minutes before or 30 minutes after the designated time.
14. Perform hand hygiene and put on PPE, if indicated.	Hand hygiene and PPE prevent the spread of microorganisms. PPE is required based on transmission precautions.
15. **Identify the patient. Compare the information with the eMAR/MAR. The patient should be identified using at least two of the following methods (The Joint Commission, 2018):**	Identifying the patient ensures the right patient receives the medications and helps prevent errors. The patient's room number or physical location is not used as an identifier (The Joint Commission, 2018). Replace the identification band if it is missing or inaccurate in any way.
a. Check the name on the patient's identification band.	This requires a response from the patient, but illness and strange surroundings often cause patients to be confused.
b. Check the identification number on the patient's identification band.	
c. Check the birth date on the patient's identification band.	
d. Ask the patient to state his or her name and birth date, based on facility policy.	
16. Close the door to the room or pull the bedside curtain.	This provides patient privacy.
17. **Complete necessary assessments before administering medications. Check the patient's allergy bracelet or ask the patient about allergies. Explain the purpose and action of the medication to the patient.**	Assessment is a prerequisite to administration of medications. Explanation provides rationale, increases knowledge, and reduces anxiety.

ACTION	**RATIONALE**
18. Scan the patient's bar code on the identification band, if required (Figure 1).	Provides an additional check to ensure that the medication is given to the right patient.

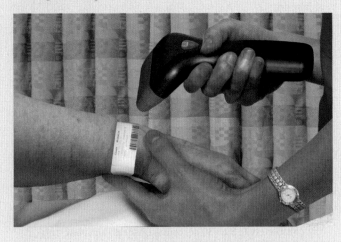

FIGURE 1. Scanning bar code on patient's identification bracelet. (*Photo by B. Proud.*)

ACTION	**RATIONALE**
19. **Based on facility policy, the third check of the label may occur at this point. If so, recheck the labels with the eMAR/MAR before administering the medications to the patient.**	Many facilities require the *third* check to occur at the bedside, after identifying the patient and before administration. If facility policy directs the *third* check at this time, this *third* check ensures accuracy and helps to prevent errors.
20. Perform hand hygiene. Put on gloves.	Hand hygiene prevents the spread of microorganisms. Gloves prevent contact with blood and body fluids.
21. Remove the cap from the syringe or insulin cartridge (Figure 2). Attach sterile tubing to the syringe or insulin cartridge. Open the pump and place the syringe or cartridge in compartment according to manufacturer's directions (Figure 3). Close the pump.	Tubing must be attached correctly and syringe must be placed in pump correctly for insulin delivery.

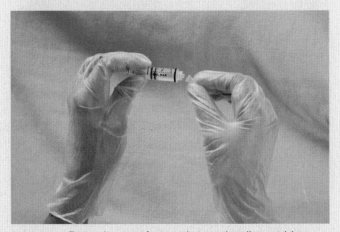

FIGURE 2. Removing cap from syringe or insulin cartridge.

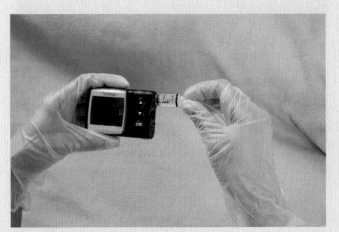

FIGURE 3. Placing syringe or cartridge in compartment according to manufacturer's directions.

(*continued*)

Skill 9 ▶ Administering a Continuous Subcutaneous Infusion: Applying an Insulin Pump *(continued)*

ACTION	RATIONALE
22. Initiate priming of the tubing, according to manufacturer's directions. Program the pump according to manufacturer's recommendations following primary care provider's orders (Figure 4). **Check for any bubbles in the tubing.**	Removing all the air from the tubing and correct programming of pump ensures the patient receives the correct dose of insulin.
23. Activate the delivery device. Place the needle between prongs of the insertion device with the sharp edge facing out. Push insertion set down until a click is heard.	To ensure correct placement of insulin pump needle, an insertion device must be used.
24. Select an appropriate administration site.	Appropriate site prevents injury.
25. Assist the patient to the appropriate position for the site chosen. Drape, as needed, to expose only site area to be used.	Appropriate site prevents injury. Draping maintains privacy and warmth.
26. **Identify the appropriate landmarks for the site chosen.**	Good visualization is necessary to establish the correct site location and to avoid tissue damage.
27. Cleanse area around injection site with antimicrobial swab (Figure 5). Use a firm, circular motion while moving outward from insertion site. Allow antiseptic to dry.	Pathogens on the skin can be forced into the tissues by the needle. Moving from the center outward prevents contamination of the site. Allowing the antimicrobial solution to dry completely (15 to 30 seconds) ensures complete antimicrobial effectiveness (Harper, 2014), and prevents introducing alcohol into the tissue, which can be irritating and uncomfortable.

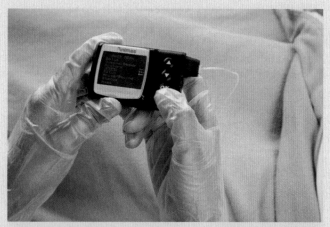

FIGURE 4. Programming pump according to manufacturer's recommendations following primary care provider's orders.

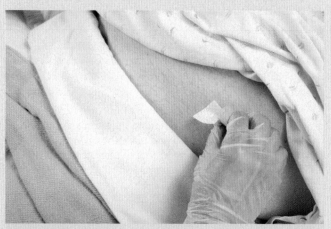

FIGURE 5. Cleansing area around injection site with antimicrobial swab.

ACTION	RATIONALE
28. Remove paper from adhesive backing. Remove the needle guard. Pinch skin at insertion site, press insertion device on site, and press release button to insert needle. Remove triggering device. Alternatively, if a needle was used to introduce a subcutaneous catheter and then withdrawn, engage the safety shield or needle guard.	To ensure delivery of insulin into subcutaneous tissue, a skin fold is made with a pinch *before* insertion of the medication. Safety shield or needle guard prevents accidental needlestick.
29. Apply sterile occlusive dressing over the insertion site, if not part of the insertion device. Attach the pump to patient's clothing, as desired (Figure 6).	Dressing prevents contamination of site. Pump can be dislodged easily if not attached securely to patient.
30. Assist the patient to a position of comfort.	This provides for the well-being of the patient.
31. If a needle was used to introduce a subcutaneous catheter and then withdrawn, discard the needle and syringe in the appropriate receptacle.	Proper disposal of the needle prevents injury.

ACTION	RATIONALE

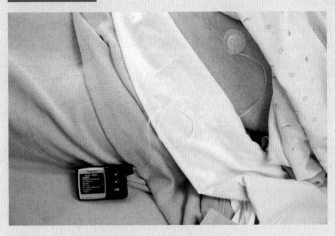

FIGURE 6. Insulin pump in place.

32. Remove gloves and additional PPE, if used. Perform hand hygiene.

Proper removal of PPE reduces the risk for infection transmission and contamination of other items. Hand hygiene prevents the spread of microorganisms.

33. Document the administration of the medication immediately after administration. See Documentation section below.

Timely documentation helps to ensure patient safety.

34. Evaluate the patient's response to the medication within the appropriate time frame. Monitor the patient's blood glucose levels, as appropriate, or as ordered.

Patient needs to be evaluated to ensure that the pump is delivering the drug appropriately. The patient needs to be evaluated for therapeutic and adverse effects from the medication.

EVALUATION

The expected outcomes have been met when the device has been applied successfully; the medication is administered correctly; the patient experiences the intended effect of the medication; the patient understands the rationale for the pump use and mechanism of action; the patient's skin remains intact; and the patient does not experience unstable blood glucose levels or adverse effect.

DOCUMENTATION

Guidelines

Document the application of the pump, the type of insulin used, pump settings, insertion site, and any teaching done with the patient on the eMAR/MAR or record using the required format, including date, time, and the site of administration, immediately after administration. If using a bar-code system, medication administration is automatically recorded when the bar code is scanned. PRN medications require documentation of the reason for administration. Prompt recording avoids the possibility of accidentally repeating the administration of the drug. If the drug was refused or omitted, record this in the appropriate area on the medication record and notify the primary care provider. This verifies the reason medication was omitted and ensures that health care personnel providing care for the patient are aware of the occurrence.

Sample Documentation

> 9/22/20 1000 Insulin pump inserted by patient on left upper quadrant of abdomen with minimal assistance. Pump filled with 300 units (3 mL) of lispro insulin. Rate set at 1 unit per hour. Patient verbalizes desire to apply pump without assistance when site next changed.
>
> —B. Clapp, RN

(*continued*)

Skill 9 ▶ Administering a Continuous Subcutaneous Infusion: Applying an Insulin Pump *(continued)*

UNEXPECTED SITUATIONS AND ASSOCIATED INTERVENTIONS

- *After the pump is attached to the patient, a large amount of air is noted in tubing:* Remove the pump from patient. Obtain new sterile tubing with insertion needle. Prime the tubing and reinsert.
- *Patient must rotate site more frequently than every 2 to 3 days due to insulin usage:* Check manufacturer's recommendations. Most pumps are initially set in a smaller mode but can be changed for a larger amount of insulin delivery.
- *Patient is refusing to rotate site at least every 3 days:* Inform the patient that absorption of medication decreases after 3 days, which may increase his or her need for insulin. Rotating sites prevents this decrease in absorption from developing. In addition, site rotation reduces risk of infection at the site.
- *You note that the insertion site is now erythematous:* Remove the stylet, obtain a new pump setup, and insert at a different site at least 1 in from old site.
- *Occlusive dressing will not stick due to perspiration:* Apply deodorant around insertion site but not over insertion site. Alternatively, apply skin barrier around insertion site but not over insertion site.

SPECIAL CONSIDERATIONS

General Considerations

- Assess infusion site areas routinely for inflammation, allergic reactions, infection, and lipodystrophy.
- Good hygiene and frequent catheter site changes reduce the risk of site complications. Change catheter site every 2 to 3 days.
- Contact dermatitis is sometimes a problem at the catheter site area. The primary care provider may order topical antibiotics, aloe, vitamin E, or corticosteroids to treat a contact dermatitis.
- Insulin self-administered by the patient through the insulin pump should be communicated to the nurse at the time of administration. This allows for accurate documentation of insulin requirements.
- Ongoing assessment is an important part of nursing care for both evaluation of patient response to administered medications and early detection of adverse reactions. If an adverse effect is suspected, withhold further medication doses and notify the patient's primary care provider. Additional intervention is based on type of reaction and patient assessment.

Home Care Considerations

- Encourage patients to consult the policies of their local government regarding contaminated and sharps waste disposal. Depending on local requirements, patients may dispose of needles and syringes in a hard, plastic container. Liquid detergent or liquid fabric softener containers are good choices. Never use glass containers.

EVIDENCE FOR PRACTICE ▶

CONTINUOUS SUBCUTANEOUS INSULIN INFUSION (CSII)

American Association of Diabetes Educators (AADE). (2014). AADE White paper. Continuous subcutaneous insulin infusion (CSII). Retrieved https://www.diabeteseducator.org/docs/default-source/legacy-docs/_resources/pdf/publications/csii_pentulimate.pdf?sfvrsn=2

This white paper outlines critical topics to be covered when teaching patients and families or significant other about insulin pump therapy. These guidelines are directed to diabetes nurse educators, but provide best-practice guidelines for all nurses caring for patients with diabetes considering or using continuous subcutaneous insulin infusion (CSII).

Skill 10 ▶ Administering Medications by Intravenous Bolus or Push Through an Intravenous Infusion

A medication can be administered via the **intravenous (IV) route** as an IV bolus or push through a venous access device being used for continuous infusion of fluid. This involves a single injection of a concentrated solution directly into an IV access. Drugs given by IV push are used for intermittent dosing or to treat emergencies. The drug is administered at the rate recommended by the manufacturer, supported by evidence in peer-reviewed biomedical literature, or in accordance with approved institutional guidelines (Institute for Safe Medication Practices, 2015, p. 13). Confirm exact administration times by consulting a drug reference, package insert, or a pharmacist.

DELEGATION CONSIDERATIONS	The administration of medications by intravenous bolus is not delegated to nursing assistive personnel (NAP) or to unlicensed assistive personnel (UAP). Depending on the state's nurse practice act and the organization's policies and procedures, the administration of specified intravenous medications in some settings may be delegated to licensed practical/vocational nurses (LPN/LVNs) who have received appropriate training. The decision to delegate must be based on careful analysis of the patient's needs and circumstances, as well as the qualifications of the person to whom the task is being delegated.
EQUIPMENT	• Antimicrobial swab • Watch or clock with second hand • Disposable gloves • Additional PPE, as indicated • Prescribed medication • 2 – Normal saline flushes prepared in a syringe (3 to 10 mL) according to facility policy • Passive disinfection caps (based on facility policy) • Syringe with a needleless device or 23- to 25-gauge, 1-in needle (follow facility policy) • Electronic Medication Administration Record (eMAR) or Medication Administration Record (MAR)
ASSESSMENT	Assess the appropriateness of the drug for the patient. Review medical history, allergy, assessment, and laboratory data that may influence drug administration. Check the expiration date before administering the medication. Assess the compatibility of the ordered medication and the IV fluid. Assess the patient's IV site for signs of any complications. Assess the patient's knowledge of the medication. If the patient has a knowledge deficit about the medication, this may be the appropriate time to begin education about the medication. If the medication may affect the patient's vital signs, assess them before administration. If the medication is for pain relief, assess the patient's pain before and after administration. Verify the patient's name, dose, route, and time of administration.
NURSING DIAGNOSIS	Determine related factors for the nursing diagnoses based on the patient's current status. Appropriate nursing diagnoses may include: • Risk for injury • Risk for allergy reaction • Risk for infection
OUTCOME IDENTIFICATION AND PLANNING	The expected outcome to achieve is that the medication is given safely via the IV route and the patient experiences the intended effect of the medication. Other outcomes that may be appropriate include the following: the patient experiences no adverse effects; and the patient understands and complies with the medication regimen.

(continued)

Skill 10 ▸ Administering Medications by Intravenous Bolus or Push Through an Intravenous Infusion *(continued)*

IMPLEMENTATION

ACTION	RATIONALE
1. Gather equipment. Check medication order against the original order in the medical record, according to facility policy. Clarify any inconsistencies. Check the patient's health record for allergies. Check a drug resource to clarify whether the medication needs to be diluted before administration. Check the administration rate.	This comparison helps to identify errors that may have occurred when orders were transcribed. The primary care provider's order or prescription is the legal record of medication orders for each facility. Compatibility of medication and solution prevents complications. Delivers the correct dose of medication as prescribed.
2. Know the actions, special nursing considerations, safe dose ranges, purpose of administration, and adverse effects of the medications to be administered. Consider the appropriateness of the medication for this patient.	This knowledge aids the nurse in evaluating the therapeutic effect of the medication in relation to the patient's disorder and can also be used to educate the patient about the medication.
3. Perform hand hygiene.	Hand hygiene prevents the spread of microorganisms.
4. Move the medication supply system to the outside of the patient's room or prepare for administration at the medication supply system in the medication area. Alternatively, access the medication administration supply system at or inside the patient's room.	Organization facilitates error-free administration and saves time.
5. Unlock the medication supply system or drawer. Enter pass code and scan employee identification, if required.	Locking the medication supply system or drawer safeguards each patient's medication supply. Facility accrediting organizations require medication supply systems to be locked when not in use. Entering pass code and scanning ID allows only authorized users into the system and identifies the user for documentation by the computer.
6. **Prepare medication for one patient at a time.**	This prevents errors in medication administration.
7. Read the eMAR/MAR and select the proper medication from the medication supply system or the patient's medication drawer.	This is the *first* check of the label.
8. Compare the label with the eMAR/MAR. Check expiration dates and perform calculations, if necessary. Scan the bar code on the package, if required.	This is the *second* check of the label. Verify calculations with another nurse to ensure safety, if necessary.
9. If necessary, withdraw medication from an ampule or vial as described in Skills 3 and 4.	
10. **Depending on facility policy, the third check of the label may occur at this point. If so, when all medications for one patient have been prepared, recheck the labels with the eMAR/MAR before taking the medications to the patient. However, many facilities require the third check to occur at the bedside, after identifying the patient.**	This *third* check ensures accuracy and helps to prevent errors. *Note:* Many facilities require the *third* check to occur at the bedside, after identifying the patient and before administration.
11. **Lock the medication supply system before leaving it.**	Locking the medication supply system or drawer safeguards the patient's medication supply. Facility accrediting organizations require medication supply systems to be locked when not in use.
12. Transport medications and equipment to the patient's bedside carefully, and keep the medications in sight at all times.	Careful handling and close observation prevent accidental or deliberate disarrangement of medications. Having equipment available saves time and facilitates performance of the task.
13. **Ensure that the patient receives the medications at the correct time.**	Check facility policy, which may allow for administration within a period of 30 minutes before or 30 minutes after the designated time.

ACTION

14. Perform hand hygiene and put on PPE, if indicated.

15. **Identify the patient. Compare the information with the eMAR/MAR. The patient should be identified using at least two of the following methods (The Joint Commission, 2018):**

   a. Check the name on the patient's identification band.

   b. Check the identification number on the patient's identification band.

   c. Check the birth date on the patient's identification band.

   d. Ask the patient to state his or her name and birth date, based on facility policy.

16. Close the door to the room or pull the bedside curtain.

17. **Complete necessary assessments before administering medications. Check the patient's allergy bracelet or ask the patient about allergies. Explain the purpose and action of the medication to the patient.**

18. Scan the patient's bar code on the identification band, if required.

19. **Based on facility policy, the third check of the label may occur at this point. If so, recheck the label with the eMAR/MAR before administering the medications to the patient.**

20. Assess IV site for presence of inflammation or infiltration or other signs of complications.

21. If IV infusion is being administered via an infusion pump, pause the pump.

22. Put on clean gloves.

23. Select injection port on the administration set that is closest to the patient. Close the clamp on the administration set immediately above the injection port (Figure 1). Do not disconnect the administration set from the venous access device hub (INS, 2016a).

RATIONALE

Hand hygiene and PPE prevent the spread of microorganisms. PPE is required based on transmission precautions.

Identifying the patient ensures the right patient receives the medications and helps prevent errors. The patient's room number or physical location is not used as an identifier (The Joint Commission, 2018). Replace the identification band if it is missing or inaccurate in any way.

This requires a response from the patient, but illness and strange surroundings often cause patients to be confused.

This provides patient privacy.

Assessment is a prerequisite to administration of medications. Explanation provides rationale, increases knowledge, and reduces anxiety.

Provides an additional check to ensure that the medication is given to the right patient.

Many facilities require the *third* check to occur at the bedside, after identifying the patient and before administration. If facility policy directs the *third* check at this time, this *third* check ensures accuracy and helps to prevent errors.

IV medication must be given directly into a vein for safe administration.

Pausing prevents infusion of fluid during bolus administration and activation of pump occlusion alarms.

Gloves prevent contact with blood and body fluids.

Using port closest to the needle insertion site minimizes dilution of medication. Closing of clamp immediately above access port ensures medication is administered to the patient and prevents medication from backing up tubing.

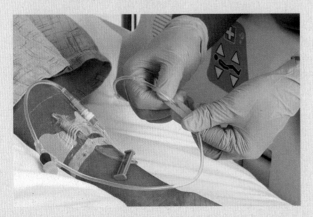

FIGURE 1. Closing the clamp on the administration set.

(*continued*)

Skill 10 ▶ Administering Medications by Intravenous Bolus or Push Through an Intravenous Infusion *(continued)*

ACTION	RATIONALE
24. Remove the passive disinfection cap from the needleless connector or end cap on the infusion set injection port (Figure 2). Alternatively, if a passive disinfection cap is not in place, use an antimicrobial swab to vigorously scrub the needleless connector or end cap on the injection port and allow to dry.	Passive disinfection caps contain an antiseptic-impregnated sponge that dispenses the antiseptic over the connector's top and threads, and protects the hub from contamination by touch or airborne sources (Stango Runyan, Stern, Macri, & Vacca, 2014). Venous access device entry points, end-caps, and needleless connectors must be vigorously scrubbed and disinfected prior to each access to reduce the risk for introduction of microorganisms and prevent venous access device-related infection (Frimpong, Caguioa, & Octavo, 2015; Harper, 2014; INS, 2016b; The Joint Commission, 2018; Loveday et al., 2014). Friction is needed to physically remove microorganisms from the top, sides, and threads of the needleless connector or end cap. Allow the antiseptic to dry completely (15 to 30 seconds) to ensure complete effectiveness (Harper).
25. Uncap saline flush syringe. Insert the saline flush syringe into the needleless connector or end cap on the injection port on the administration tubing (Figure 3).	Assessing patency of venous access device is necessary to ensure intravenous administration of the medication.

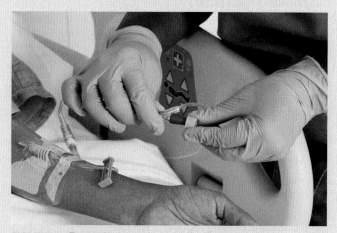

FIGURE 2. Removing the passive disinfection cap.

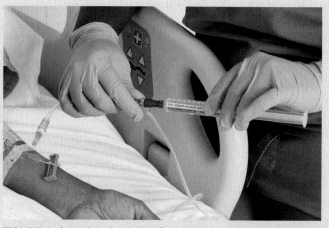

FIGURE 3. Inserting the saline flush syringe into the injection port.

26. Pull back on the syringe plunger to aspirate the catheter for positive blood return (Figure 4). If positive, instill the solution over 1 minute or flush the line according to facility policy. Remove syringe.	Positive blood return confirms patency before administration of medications and solutions (INS, 2016b). Flushing without incident ensures patency of the IV line and administration of medication into the bloodstream.

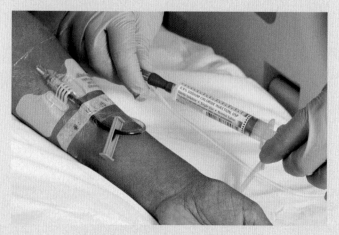

FIGURE 4. Pulling back on plunger to check blood return.

ACTION

27. Use an antimicrobial swab to vigorously scrub the needle-less connector or end cap on the injection port and allow to dry.

28. Uncap the medication syringe. Insert the medication syringe into the needleless connector or end cap on the injection port. Using a watch or clock with a second-hand to time the rate, **inject the medication at the recommended rate (Figure 5).**

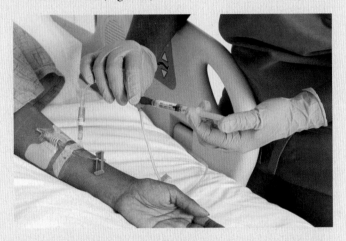

29. While administering the medication, observe the infusion site and assess patient for any adverse reaction. If signs of adverse reaction occur, stop infusion immediately and notify the primary health provider.

30. Detach the medication syringe. Use a new antimicrobial swab to vigorously scrub the needleless connector or end cap on the injection port, and allow to dry. Uncap the second saline flush syringe. Insert the saline flush syringe into the needleless connector or end cap on injection port. Instill the flush solution at the same rate as the administered medication (INS, 2016a).

31. Remove the flush syringe. Unclamp the administration set above the injection port.

RATIONALE

Venous access device entry points, end-caps, and needleless connectors must be vigorously scrubbed and disinfected prior to each access to reduce the risk for introduction of microorganisms and prevent venous access device-related infection (Frimpong et al., 2015; Harper, 2014; INS, 2016b; The Joint Commission, 2018; Loveday et al., 2014). Friction is needed to physically remove microorganisms from the top, sides, and threads of the needleless connector or end cap. Allow the antiseptic to dry completely (15 to 30 seconds) to ensure complete effectiveness (Harper, 2014).

This delivers the correct amount of medication at the proper interval.

FIGURE 5. Injecting medication at the recommended rate.

Signs of adverse reaction, such as peripheral IV infiltration, rash or itching, or pain at the infusion, necessitate stopping of administration of the drug (INS, 2016a).

Venous access device entry points, end-caps, and needleless connectors must be vigorously scrubbed and disinfected prior to each access to reduce the risk for introduction of microorganisms and prevent venous access device-related infection (Frimpong et al., 2015; Harper, 2014; INS, 2016b; The Joint Commission, 2018; Loveday et al., 2014). Friction is needed to physically remove microorganisms from the top, sides, and threads of the needleless connector or end cap. Allow the antiseptic to dry completely (15 to 30 seconds) to ensure complete effectiveness (Harper). Flushing after medication administration ensure the entire drug dose has been cleared from the extension tubing on the venous access device or from the infusion system and prevents precipitation due to solution/medication incompatibility (INS, 2016a).

Clamping prevents air from entering the extension set on a capped venous access device. Unclamping the administration set allows for resumption of the continuous intravenous infusion.

(continued)

Skill 10 ▶ Administering Medications by Intravenous Bolus or Push Through an Intravenous Infusion *(continued)*

ACTION

32. Using an antimicrobial swab, vigorously scrub the needleless connector or end cap on the extension tubing and allow to dry. Attach a passive disinfection cap to the needleless connector or end cap on the extension tubing or the injection port on the administration set (Figure 6).

RATIONALE

Venous access device entry points, end-caps, and needleless connectors must be vigorously scrubbed and disinfected prior to each access to reduce the risk for introduction of microorganisms and prevent venous access device-related infection (Frimpong et al., 2015; Harper, 2014; INS, 2016b; The Joint Commission, 2018; Loveday et al., 2014). Friction is needed to physically remove microorganisms from the top, sides, and threads of the needleless connector or end cap. Allow the antiseptic to dry completely (15 to 30 seconds) to ensure complete effectiveness (Harper, 2014). Passive disinfection caps contain an antiseptic-impregnated sponge that dispenses the antiseptic over the connector's top and threads, and protect the hub from contamination by touch or airborne sources (Stango et al., 2014).

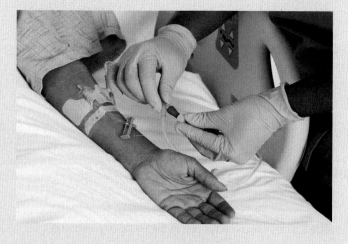

FIGURE 6. Attaching a passive disinfection cap.

33. Restart the infusion pump and check IV fluid infusion rate.

Restarting infusion pump resumes prescribed continuous infusion of fluid. Checking IV fluid infusion rate assures accuracy in administration.

34. Discard the syringe in the appropriate receptacle.

Proper disposal prevents injury and spread of microorganisms.

35. Remove gloves and additional PPE, if used. Perform hand hygiene.

Proper removal of PPE reduces the risk for infection transmission and contamination of other items. Hand hygiene prevents the spread of microorganisms.

36. Document the administration of the medication immediately after administration. See Documentation section below.

Timely documentation helps to ensure patient safety.

37. Evaluate the patient's response to the medication within the appropriate time frame.

The patient needs to be evaluated for therapeutic and adverse effects from the medication.

EVALUATION

The expected outcomes have been met when the medication has been given safely via the IV route and the patient experiences the intended effect of the medication; the patient experiences no adverse effects; and the patient understands and complies with the medication regimen.

DOCUMENTATION

Guidelines

Document the administration of the medication immediately after administration, including date, time, dose, route of administration, site of administration, and rate of administration on the eMAR/MAR or record using the required format. If using a bar-code system, medication administration is automatically recorded when the bar code is scanned. PRN medications require documentation of the reason for administration. Prompt recording avoids the possibility of accidentally repeating the administration of the drug. If the drug was refused or omitted, record this in the appropriate area on the medication record and notify the primary care provider. This verifies the reason medication was omitted and ensures that health care personnel providing care for the patient are aware of the occurrence.

UNEXPECTED SITUATIONS AND ASSOCIATED INTERVENTIONS

- *Upon assessing the IV site before administering medication, no blood return is aspirated:* If IV appears patent, without signs of infiltration, and IV fluid infuses without difficulty, proceed with administration. Observe closely for signs and symptoms of infiltration during and after administration.
- *Upon assessing the patient's IV site before administering medication, you note that IV has infiltrated:* Stop IV fluid and remove IV from extremity. Restart IV in a different location. Continue to monitor new IV site as medication is administered.
- *While administering medication, you note a cloudy, white substance forming in the IV tubing:* Stop administering medication. Clamp IV at the site nearest to the patient. Change administration tubing and restart infusion. Check literature or consult pharmacist regarding compatibility of medication and IV fluid.
- *While you are administering the medication, the patient begins to complain of pain at the IV site:* Stop medication. Assess IV site for any signs of infiltration or phlebitis. Flush the IV with normal saline to check for patency. If the IV site appears within normal limits, resume medication administration at a slower rate.

SPECIAL CONSIDERATIONS

- Do not withdraw IV push medications from commercially available, cartridge-type syringes into another syringe for administration. Using the cartridge as a vial can lead to contamination and/or dosing errors, drug mix-ups, and other medication errors (ISMP, 2015, p. 11).
- Do not dilute or reconstitute IV push medications by drawing up the contents into a commercially available, prefilled flush syringe of 0.9% sodium chloride. These devices have been approved for flushing of vascular access devices, but have not been approved for the reconstitution, dilution, and/or subsequent administration of IV push medications (ISMP, 2015, p. 11).
- Appropriately label all clinician-prepared syringes of IV push medications or solutions, unless the medication or solution is prepared at the patient's bedside and is immediately administered to the patient (ISMP, 2015, p. 12).
- If the IV is a small gauge (22- to 24-gauge) placed in a small vein, a blood return may not occur even if IV is intact. Also, the patient may complain of stinging and pain at the site while medication is being administered due to irritation of vein. Slowing the rate of administration may relieve discomfort.
- Ongoing assessment is an important part of nursing care for both evaluation of patient response to administered medications and early detection of adverse drug reactions. If an adverse effect is suspected, withhold further medication doses and notify the patient's primary care provider. Additional intervention is based on type of reaction and patient assessment.

EVIDENCE FOR PRACTICE ▶

INFUSION NURSING STANDARDS OF PRACTICE

Infusion Nurses Society (INS). (2016b). Infusion therapy. Standards of practice. *Journal of Infusion Nursing, 39*(Suppl 1), S1–S159.

The Infusion Nurses Society is recognized as the global authority in infusion therapy. The *Infusion Nursing Standards of Practice* is an evidence-based document, providing guidelines for nurses related to infusion therapy for use in all patient settings and addressing all patient populations.

(continued)

Skill 10 ▶ Administering Medications by Intravenous Bolus or Push Through an Intravenous Infusion *(continued)*

EVIDENCE FOR PRACTICE ▶	**INFUSION NURSING POLICIES AND PROCEDURES FOR INFUSION THERAPY** Infusion Nurses Society (INS). (2016a). *Policies and procedures for infusion therapy* (5th ed.). Norwood, MA: Author. The Infusion Nurses Society is recognized as the global authority in infusion therapy. The *Infusion Nursing Standards of Practice* is an evidence-based document, providing policies and step-by-step procedures for nurses related to infusion therapy for use in all patient settings and addressing all patient populations.

Skill 11 ▶ Administering a Piggyback Intermittent Intravenous Infusion of Medication

Medications can be administered by intermittent intravenous infusion. The drug is mixed with a small amount of the IV solution, such as 50 to 100 mL, and administered over a short period at the prescribed interval (e.g., every 8 hours). The administration is most often performed using an electronic infusion device (IV or infusion pump), which requires the nurse to program the infusion rate into the pump. Smart pumps are intravenous infusion devices that are used to administer intermittent infusions and provide computerized dose error-reduction software with IV therapy libraries and corresponding administration rate limits (Harding, 2013). Smart pumps are used in the majority (77%) of hospital settings in the United States (Pedersen, Schneider & Scheckelhoff, 2013). Administration of an intermittent infusion may also be achieved by gravity infusion, which requires the nurse to calculate the infusion rate in drops per minute. The best practice, however, is to use an electronic infusion device.

Although newer infusion pumps allow for more flexibly (including concurrent programming of primary and secondary/piggyback lines), some intravenous piggyback delivery systems still require the container with the intermittent or additive solution to be placed higher than the primary solution container. An extension hook provided by the manufacturer provides for easy lowering of the main IV container. The port on the primary IV line has a back-check valve that automatically stops the flow of the primary solution, allowing the secondary or piggyback solution to flow when connected. Because manufacturers' designs vary, it is important to check the directions carefully for the systems used in the facility.

DELEGATION CONSIDERATIONS

The administration of medications by intermittent IV infusion is not delegated to nursing assistive personnel (NAP) or to unlicensed assistive personnel (UAP). Depending on the state's nurse practice act and the organization's policies and procedures, the administration of specified IV medications in some settings may be delegated to licensed practical/vocational nurses (LPN/LVNs) who have received appropriate training. The decision to delegate must be based on careful analysis of the patient's needs and circumstances, as well as the qualifications of the person to whom the task is being delegated.

EQUIPMENT

- Medication prepared in labeled small-volume bag
- Short secondary infusion tubing
- Infusion pump
- Antimicrobial swab
- Needleless connector, if required, based on facility procedure
- Metal or plastic hook
- IV pole

- Watch or clock with a second hand (gravity infusion)
- Date label for tubing
- Electronic Medication Administration Record (eMAR) or Medication Administration Record (MAR)
- PPE, as indicated

ASSESSMENT

Assess the appropriateness of the drug for the patient. Review medical history, allergy, assessment, and laboratory data that may influence drug administration. Check the expiration date before administering the medication. **Assess the compatibility of the ordered medication, diluent, and the infusing IV fluid.** Assess the patient's IV site for signs of any complications. Assess the patient's knowledge of the medication. If the patient has a knowledge deficit about the medication, this may be the appropriate time to begin education about the medication. If the medication may affect the patient's vital signs, assess them before administration. Verify patient name, dose, route, and time of administration.

NURSING DIAGNOSIS

Determine related factors for the nursing diagnoses based on the patient's current status. Appropriate nursing diagnoses include:

- Risk for allergy reaction
- Risk for infection
- Risk for injury

OUTCOME IDENTIFICATION AND PLANNING

The expected outcome to achieve is that the medication is delivered via the intravenous route and the patient experiences the intended effect of the medication. Other outcomes that may be appropriate include the following: the patient experiences no adverse effects; and the patient understands and complies with the medication regimen.

IMPLEMENTATION

ACTION	RATIONALE
1. Gather equipment. Check each medication order against the original order in the health record, according to facility policy. Clarify any inconsistencies. Check the patient's health record for allergies.	This comparison helps to identify errors that may have occurred when orders were transcribed. The primary care provider's order or prescription is the legal record of medication orders for each facility.
2. Know the actions, special nursing considerations, safe dose ranges, purpose of administration, and adverse effects of the medications to be administered. Consider the appropriateness of the medication for this patient. **Assess the compatibility of the ordered medication, diluent, and the infusing IV fluid.**	This knowledge aids the nurse in evaluating the therapeutic effect of the medication in relation to the patient's disorder and can also be used to educate the patient about the medication. Compatibility of medication and solutions prevents complications.
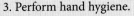3. Perform hand hygiene.	Hand hygiene prevents the spread of microorganisms.
4. Move the medication supply system to the outside of the patient's room or prepare for administration at the medication supply system in the medication area. Alternatively, access the medication administration supply system at or inside the patient's room.	Organization facilitates error-free administration and saves time.

(continued)

Skill 11 ▸ Administering a Piggyback Intermittent Intravenous Infusion of Medication *(continued)*

ACTION	RATIONALE
5. Unlock the medication supply system or drawer. Enter pass code and scan employee identification, if required.	Locking the medication supply system or drawer safeguards each patient's medication supply. Facility accrediting organizations require medication supply systems to be locked when not in use. Entering pass code and scanning ID allows only authorized users into the system and identifies the user for documentation by the computer.
6. **Prepare medications for one patient at a time.**	This prevents errors in medication administration.
7. Read the eMAR/MAR and select the proper medication from the medication supply system or the patient's medication drawer.	This is the *first* check of the label.
8. Compare the label with the eMAR/MAR. Check expiration dates. Confirm the prescribed or appropriate infusion rate. Calculate the drip rate if using a gravity system. Scan the bar code on the package, if required.	This is the *second* check of the label. Verify calculations with another nurse to ensure safety, if necessary. Infusing medication at an appropriate rate prevents injury.
9. **Depending on facility policy, the third check of the label may occur at this point. If so, when all medications for one patient have been prepared, recheck the labels with the eMAR/MAR before taking the medications to the patient. However, many facilities require the third check to occur at the bedside, after identifying the patient.**	This *third* check ensures accuracy and helps to prevent errors. *Note:* Many facilities require the *third* check to occur at the bedside, after identifying the patient and before administration.
10. **Lock the medication supply system before leaving it.**	Locking the medication supply system or drawer safeguards the patient's medication supply. Facility accrediting organizations require medication supply systems to be locked when not in use.
11. Transport medications to the patient's bedside carefully, and keep the medications in sight at all times.	Careful handling and close observation prevent accidental or deliberate disarrangement of medications.
12. **Ensure that the patient receives the medications at the correct time.**	Check facility policy, which may allow for administration within a period of 30 minutes before or 30 minutes after the designated time.
13. Perform hand hygiene and put on PPE, if indicated.	Hand hygiene and PPE prevent the spread of microorganisms. PPE is required based on transmission precautions.
14. **Identify the patient. Compare the information with the eMAR/MAR. The patient should be identified using at least two of the following methods (The Joint Commission, 2018):**	Identifying the patient ensures the right patient receives the medications and helps prevent errors. The patient's room number or physical location is not used as an identifier (The Joint Commission, 2018). Replace the identification band if it is missing or inaccurate in any way.
a. Check the name on the patient's identification band. b. Check the identification number on the patient's identification band. c. Check the birth date on the patient's identification band. d. Ask the patient to state his or her name and birth date, based on facility policy.	This requires a response from the patient, but illness and strange surroundings often cause patients to be confused.
15. Close the door to the room or pull the bedside curtain.	This provides patient privacy.
16. **Complete necessary assessments before administering medications. Check the patient's allergy bracelet or ask the patient about allergies. Explain the purpose and action of the medication to the patient.**	Assessment is a prerequisite to administration of medications. Explanation provides rationale, increases knowledge, and reduces anxiety.

ACTION	RATIONALE
17. Scan the patient's bar code on the identification band, if required.	Scanning provides an additional check to ensure that the medication is given to the right patient.
18. **Based on facility policy, the third check of the label may occur at this point. If so, recheck the labels with the eMAR/MAR before administering the medications to the patient.**	Many facilities require the *third* check to occur at the bedside, after identifying the patient and before administration. If facility policy directs the *third* check at this time, this *third* check ensures accuracy and helps to prevent errors.
19. Assess the IV site for the presence of complications.	IV medication must be given directly into a vein for safe administration.
20. Close the clamp on the short secondary infusion tubing. Using aseptic technique, remove the cap on the tubing spike and the cap on the port of the medication container, taking care to avoid contaminating either end.	Closing the clamp prevents fluid from entering the system until the nurse is ready. Maintaining sterility of the tubing and the medication port prevents contamination.
21. Attach infusion tubing to the medication container by inserting the tubing spike into the port with a firm push and twisting motion, taking care to avoid contaminating either end.	Maintaining sterility of tubing and medication port prevents contamination.
22. Hang piggyback container on IV pole, positioning it higher than primary IV according to manufacturer's recommendations (Figure 1). If necessary for the particular infusion pump in use, use the metal or plastic hook to lower primary IV fluid container. If using gravity infusion, primary IV fluid container must be lowered.	Position of containers influences the flow of IV fluid into the primary setup.

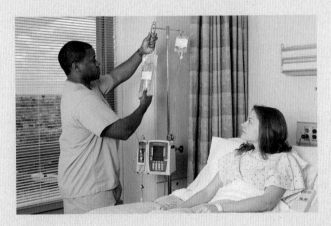

FIGURE 1. Positioning piggyback container on IV pole. (*Photo by B. Proud.*)

ACTION	RATIONALE
23. Place label on administration tubing with the current date.	Label identifies the date of first use of the tubing. Intermittent administration sets disconnected after use should be replaced every 24 hours; repeated disconnection and reconnection increases risk of contamination at the spike end, catheter hub, needleless connector, and the end of the administration set, potentially increasing the risk for catheter-related bloodstream infection (INS, 2016b)
24. Squeeze drip chamber on administration tubing and release. Fill chamber to the line or about half full. Open clamp on administration tubing and prime tubing. Close clamp. Place needleless connector on the end of the tubing, using sterile technique, if required.	This removes air from tubing and preserves the sterility of the setup.

(*continued*)

Skill 11 ▶ Administering a Piggyback Intermittent Intravenous Infusion of Medication *(continued)*

25. Remove the passive disinfection cap from the needleless connector or end cap on the infusion set injection port. Alternatively, if a passive disinfection cap is not in place, use an antimicrobial swab to vigorously scrub the access port or stopcock on the administration set above where the tubing enters the infusion pump or above the roller clamp on the primary IV infusion tubing (gravity infusion) (Figure 2).

Passive disinfection caps contain an antiseptic-impregnated sponge that dispenses the antiseptic over the connector's top and threads, and protects the hub from contamination by touch or airborne sources (Stango et al., 2014). Venous access device entry points, end-caps, and needleless connectors must be vigorously scrubbed and disinfected prior to each access to reduce the risk for introduction of microorganisms and prevent venous access device-related infection (Frimpong et al., 2015; Harper, 2014; INS, 2016b; The Joint Commission, 2018; Loveday et al., 2014). Friction is needed to physically remove microorganisms from the top, sides, and threads of the needleless connector or end cap. Allow the antiseptic to dry completely (15 to 30 seconds) to ensure complete effectiveness (Harper, 2014). Backflow valve in the primary line secondary port stops flow of primary infusion while piggyback solution is infusing. Once completed, backflow valves open and flow of primary solution resumes.

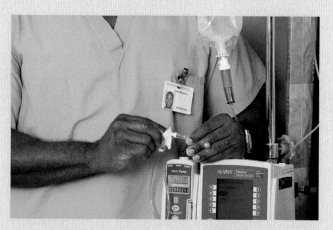

FIGURE 2. Vigorously scrubbing the access port. (*Photo by B. Proud.*)

26. Connect piggyback setup to the access port or stopcock (Figure 3). If using, turn the stopcock to the open position.

Needleless systems and stopcock setup eliminate the need for a needle and are recommended by the CDC.

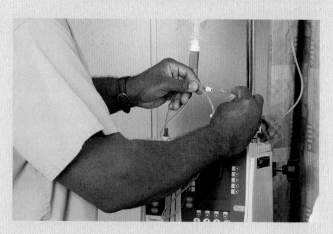

FIGURE 3. Connecting piggyback administration set to access port. (*Photo by B. Proud.*)

ACTION

27. Open clamp on the secondary infusion tubing. Set rate for secondary infusion on infusion pump and begin infusion (Figure 4). If using gravity infusion, use the roller clamp on the primary infusion tubing to regulate the flow at the prescribed delivery rate (Figure 5). Monitor medication infusion at periodic intervals.

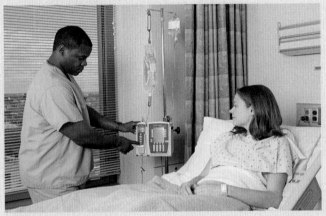

FIGURE 4. Setting rate for secondary infusion on infusion pump. (*Photo by B. Proud.*)

28. Clamp tubing on piggyback set when solution is infused. Follow facility policy regarding disposal of equipment.

29. Raise primary IV fluid container to original height. **Check primary infusion rate on infusion pump. If using gravity infusion, readjust flow rate of primary IV.**

 30. Remove PPE, if used. Perform hand hygiene.

31. Document the administration of the medication immediately after administration. See Documentation section below. Document the volume of fluid administered on the intake and output record, if necessary.

32. Evaluate the patient's response to the medication within an appropriate time frame. Monitor IV site at periodic intervals.

RATIONALE

Backflow valve in the primary line secondary port stops flow of primary infusion while piggyback solution is infusing. Once completed, backflow valves open and flow of primary solution resumes. It is important to verify the safe administration rate for each drug to prevent adverse effects.

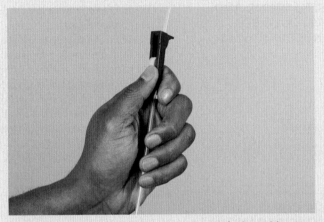

FIGURE 5. Using roller clamp on primary infusion tubing to regulate gravity flow. (*Photo by B. Proud.*)

Most facilities allow the reuse of tubing, reducing the risk for contamination. The frequency of administration set tubing changes varies.

Most infusion pumps automatically restart primary infusion at previous rate after secondary infusion is completed. If using gravity infusion, piggyback medication administration may interrupt normal flow rate of primary IV. Rate readjustment may be necessary.

Proper removal of PPE reduces the risk for infection transmission and contamination of other items. Hand hygiene prevents the spread of microorganisms.

Timely documentation helps to ensure patient safety.

The patient needs to be evaluated for therapeutic and adverse effects from the medication.

EVALUATION

The expected outcomes have been met when the medication is delivered via the intravenous route; the patient experiences the intended effect of the medication; the patient experiences no adverse effects; and the patient understands and complies with the medication regimen.

DOCUMENTATION

Guidelines

Document the administration of the medication immediately after administration, including date, time, dose, route of administration, site of administration, and rate of administration on the eMAR/MAR or record using the required format. If using a bar-code system, medication administration is

(*continued*)

Skill 11 ▶ Administering a Piggyback Intermittent Intravenous Infusion of Medication *(continued)*

automatically recorded when the bar code is scanned. PRN medications require documentation of the reason for administration. Prompt recording avoids the possibility of accidentally repeating the administration of the drug. If the drug was refused or omitted, record this in the appropriate area on the medication record and notify the primary care provider. This verifies the reason medication was omitted and ensures that health care personnel providing care for the patient are aware of the occurrence. Document the volume of fluid administered on the intake and output record, if necessary.

UNEXPECTED SITUATIONS AND ASSOCIATED INTERVENTIONS

- *Upon assessing the IV site before administering medication, you note that the IV has infiltrated:* Stop IV fluid and remove the IV from the extremity. Restart the IV in a different location. Continue to monitor the new IV site as medication is administered.
- *While administering medication, you note a cloudy, white substance forming in the IV tubing:* Stop the IV from flowing and stop administering the medication to prevent precipitate from entering the patient's circulation. Clamp the IV at the site nearest to the patient. Replace tubing on primary and secondary infusions. Check the literature regarding incompatibilities of medications before administering. Medication infusion may require a second IV site or administration through an access port closer to the IV site and flushing of tubing before and after administration.
- *While you are administering medication, the patient begins to complain of pain at the IV site:* Stop the medication. Assess the IV site for any signs of complications. Flush the IV with normal saline to check for patency. If the IV site appears within normal limits, resume medication administration at a slower rate.

SPECIAL CONSIDERATIONS

General Considerations

- An alternate way to prime the secondary tubing, particularly if administration set is in place from a previous infusion, is to "backfill" the secondary tubing. Attach the medication bag to the secondary infusion tubing. Lower the medication bag below the main IV solution container and open the clamp on the secondary infusion tubing. This allows the primary IV solution to flow up the secondary tubing to the drip chamber, "backfilling" the tubing. Allow the solution to enter the drip chamber until the drip chamber is half full. Close the clamp on the secondary tubing and hang the medication container on the IV pole. Proceed with administration by lowering the primary IV container, as described above. This "backfill" method keeps the infusion system intact, preventing both introduction of microorganisms and loss of medication when the tubing is primed. Check facility policy regarding the use of "backfilling."
- Intermittent administration sets disconnected after use should be replaced every 24 hours; repeated disconnection and reconnection increases risk of contamination at the spike end, catheter hub, needleless connector, and the end of the administration set, potentially increasing the risk for catheter-related bloodstream infection (INS, 2016b).
- Ongoing assessment is an important part of nursing care for both evaluation of patient response to administered medications and early detection of adverse reactions. If an adverse effect is suspected, withhold further medication doses and notify the patient's primary care provider. Additional intervention is based on type of reaction and patient assessment.

Infant and Child Considerations

- Infants and small children with fluid restrictions may not tolerate the added IV fluid needed for administration with piggyback systems. For these children, consider using the mini-infusion pump (see Skill 12).

EVIDENCE FOR PRACTICE ▶

INFUSION NURSING STANDARDS OF PRACTICE

Infusion Nurses Society (INS). (2016b). Infusion therapy. Standards of practice. *Journal of Infusion Nursing, 39*(Suppl 1), S1–S159.

Refer to details in Skill 10, Evidence for Practice.

EVIDENCE FOR PRACTICE ▶   **INFUSION NURSING POLICIES AND PROCEDURES FOR INFUSION THERAPY**

Infusion Nurses Society (INS). (2016a). *Policies and procedures for infusion therapy* (5th ed.). Norwood, MA: Author.

Refer to details in Skill 10, Evidence for Practice

Skill 12 ▶ Administering an Intermittent Intravenous Infusion of Medication via a Mini-Infusion Pump

Medications can be administered by intermittent intravenous infusion. The mini-infusion pump (syringe pump) for intermittent infusion is battery- or electrical-operated and allows medication mixed in a syringe to be connected to the primary line and delivered by mechanical pressure applied to the syringe plunger. Mini-infusion pumps may use a smart pump design; smart pumps are intravenous infusion devices that are used to administer intermittent infusions and provide computerized dose error-reduction software with IV therapy libraries and corresponding administration rate limits (Harding, 2013). Smart pumps are used in the majority (77%) of hospital settings in the United States (Pedersen et al., 2013).

DELEGATION CONSIDERATIONS

The administration of medications by intermittent IV infusion is not delegated to nursing assistive personnel (NAP) or to unlicensed assistive personnel (UAP). Depending on the state's nurse practice act and the organization's policies and procedures, the administration of specified IV medications in some settings may be delegated to licensed practical/vocational nurses (LPN/LVNs) who have received appropriate training. The decision to delegate must be based on careful analysis of the patient's needs and circumstances, as well as the qualifications of the person to whom the task is being delegated.

EQUIPMENT

- Medication prepared in labeled syringe
- Mini-infusion pump and tubing
- Needleless connector, if required, based on facility system
- Antimicrobial swab
- Date label for tubing
- Electronic Medication Administration Record (eMAR) or Medication Administration Record (MAR)
- PPE, as indicated

ASSESSMENT

Assess the appropriateness of the drug for the patient. Review medical history, allergy, assessment, and laboratory data that may influence drug administration. Check the expiration date before administering medication. **Assess the compatibility of the ordered medication, diluent, and the infusing IV fluid.** Assess the patient's IV site for signs of any complications. Assess the patient's knowledge of the medication. If the patient has a knowledge deficit about the medication, this may be the appropriate time to begin education about the medication. If the medication may affect the patient's vital signs, assess them before administration. Verify patient name, dose, route, and time of administration. Assess the patient's knowledge of the medication.

NURSING DIAGNOSIS

Determine related factors for the nursing diagnoses based on the patient's current status. Appropriate nursing diagnoses include:

- Risk for allergy reaction
- Risk for injury
- Risk for infection

(continued)

Skill 12 ▶ Administering an Intermittent Intravenous Infusion of Medication via a Mini-Infusion Pump *(continued)*

OUTCOME IDENTIFICATION AND PLANNING

The expected outcome is that the medication is delivered via the IV route and the patient experiences the intended effect of the medication. Other outcomes that may be appropriate include the following: the patient experiences no adverse effects; and the patient understands and complies with the medication regimen.

IMPLEMENTATION

ACTION	RATIONALE
1. Gather equipment. Check each medication order against the original order in the health record according to facility policy. Clarify any inconsistencies. Check the patient's health record for allergies.	This comparison helps to identify errors that may have occurred when orders were transcribed. The primary care provider's order or prescription is the legal record of medication orders for each facility. Compatibility of medication and solution prevents complications.
2. Know the actions, special nursing considerations, safe dose ranges, purpose of administration, and adverse effects of the medications to be administered. Consider the appropriateness of the medication for this patient. **Assess the compatibility of the ordered medication, diluent, and the infusing IV fluid.**	This knowledge aids the nurse in evaluating the therapeutic effect of the medication in relation to the patient's disorder and can also be used to educate the patient about the medication. Compatibility of medication and solutions prevents complications.
3. Perform hand hygiene.	Hand hygiene prevents the spread of microorganisms.
4. Move the medication supply system to the outside of the patient's room or prepare for administration at the medication supply system in the medication area. Alternatively, access the medication administration supply system at or inside the patient's room.	Organization facilitates error-free administration and saves time.
5. Unlock the medication supply system or drawer. Enter pass code and scan employee identification, if required.	Locking the medication supply system or drawer safeguards each patient's medication supply. Facility accrediting organizations require medication supply systems to be locked when not in use. Entering pass code and scanning ID allows only authorized users into the system and identifies the user for documentation by the computer.
6. **Prepare medications for one patient at a time.**	This prevents errors in medication administration.
7. Read the eMAR/MAR and select the proper medication from the medication supply system or the patient's medication drawer.	This is the *first* check of the label.
8. Compare the label with the eMAR/MAR. Check expiration dates. Confirm the prescribed or appropriate infusion rate. Scan the bar code on the package, if required.	This is the *second* check of the label. Verify calculations with another nurse to ensure safety, if necessary. Infusing medication at appropriate rate prevents injury.
9. **Depending on facility policy, the third check of the label may occur at this point. If so, when all medications for one patient have been prepared, recheck the labels with the eMAR/MAR before taking the medications to the patient. However, many facilities require the third check to occur at the bedside, after identifying the patient.**	This *third* check ensures accuracy and helps to prevent errors. *Note:* Many facilities require the *third* check to occur at the bedside, after identifying the patient and before administration.
10. **Lock the medication supply system before leaving it.**	Locking the medication supply system or drawer safeguards the patient's medication supply. Facility accrediting organizations require medication supply systems to be locked when not in use.

ACTION	**RATIONALE**
11. Transport medications to the patient's bedside carefully, and keep the medications in sight at all times.	Careful handling and close observation prevent accidental or deliberate disarrangement of medications.
12. **Ensure that the patient receives the medications at the correct time.**	Check facility policy, which may allow for administration within a period of 30 minutes before or 30 minutes after the designated time.
13. Perform hand hygiene and put on PPE, if indicated.	Hand hygiene and PPE prevent the spread of microorganisms. PPE is required based on transmission precautions.
14. **Identify the patient. Compare the information with the eMAR/MAR. The patient should be identified using at least two of the following methods (The Joint Commission, 2018):**	Identifying the patient ensures the right patient receives the medications and helps prevent errors. The patient's room number or physical location is not used as an identifier (The Joint Commission, 2018). Replace the identification band if it is missing or inaccurate in any way.
a. Check the name on the patient's identification band. b. Check the identification number on the patient's identification band. c. Check the birth date on the patient's identification band. d. Ask the patient to state his or her name and birth date, based on facility policy.	This requires a response from the patient, but illness and strange surroundings often cause patients to be confused.
15. Close the door to the room or pull the bedside curtain.	Provides patient privacy.
16. **Complete necessary assessments before administering medications. Check the patient's allergy bracelet or ask the patient about allergies. Explain the purpose and action of the medication to the patient.**	Assessment is a prerequisite to administration of medications. Explanation provides rationale, increases knowledge, and reduces anxiety.
17. Scan the patient's bar code on the identification band, if required.	Provides an additional check to ensure that the medication is given to the right patient.
18. **Based on facility policy, the third check of the label may occur at this point. If so, recheck the labels with the eMAR/MAR before administering the medications to the patient.**	Many facilities require the *third* check to occur at the bedside, after identifying the patient and before administration. If facility policy directs the *third* check at this time, this *third* check ensures accuracy and helps to prevent errors.
19. Assess the IV site for the presence of complications.	IV medication must be given directly into a vein for safe administration.
20. Using aseptic technique, remove the cap on the administration tubing and the cap on the medication syringe, taking care not to contaminate either end.	Maintaining sterility of tubing and medication port prevents contamination.
21. Attach administration tubing to the syringe, taking care not to contaminate either end.	Maintaining sterility of tubing and medication port prevents contamination.
22. Place label on tubing with current date.	Label identifies the date of first use of the tubing. Intermittent administration sets disconnected after use should be replaced every 24 hours; repeated disconnection and reconnection increases risk of contamination at the spike end, catheter hub, needleless connector and the end of the administration set, potential increasing the risk for catheter-related bloodstream infection (INS, 2016b).
23. Fill administration tubing (prime) with medication by applying gentle pressure to syringe plunger. Place needleless connector on the end of the tubing, if required, using sterile technique.	This removes air from tubing and maintains sterility.

(continued)

Skill 12 ▶ Administering an Intermittent Intravenous Infusion of Medication via a Mini-Infusion Pump *(continued)*

ACTION	RATIONALE
24. Insert syringe into mini-infusion pump according to manufacturer's directions (Figure 1).	Syringe must fit securely in pump apparatus for proper operation.
25. Remove the passive disinfection cap from the needleless connector or end cap on the access port on the primary IV infusion tubing, closest to the IV insertion site (Figure 2). Alternatively, if a passive disinfection cap is not in place, use an antimicrobial swab to vigorously scrub the access port or stopcock above the roller clamp on the primary IV infusion tubing, usually the port closest to the IV insertion site.	Passive disinfection caps contain an antiseptic-impregnated sponge that dispenses the antiseptic over the connector's top and threads, and protects the hub from contamination by touch or airborne sources (Stango et al., 2014). Venous access device entry points, end-caps, and needleless connectors must be vigorously scrubbed and disinfected prior to each access to reduce the risk for introduction of microorganisms and prevent venous access device-related infection (Frimpong et al., 2015; Harper, 2014; INS, 2016b; The Joint Commission, 2018; Loveday et al., 2014). Friction is needed to physically remove microorganisms from the top, sides, and threads of the needleless connector or end cap. Allow the antiseptic to dry completely (15 to 30 seconds) to ensure complete effectiveness (Harper, 2014). Proper connection allows IV medication to flow into the primary line.
26. Connect the secondary infusion to the primary infusion at the access port (Figure 3).	Allows for delivery of medication.
27. Program the mini-infusion pump to the appropriate rate and begin infusion (Figure 4). Set the alarm if recommended by the manufacturer.	Pump delivers medication at a controlled rate. Alarm is recommended for use with IV lock apparatus.

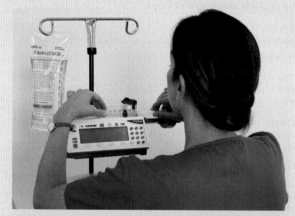

FIGURE 1. Inserting syringe into mini-infusion pump.

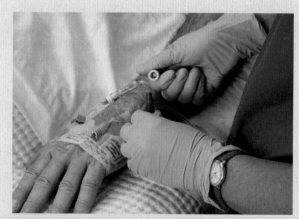

FIGURE 2. Removing the passive disinfection cap from the access port closest to IV insertion site.

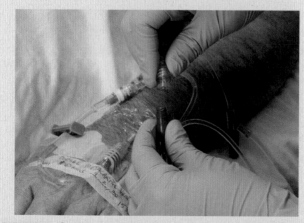

FIGURE 3. Connecting secondary infusion tubing the access port.

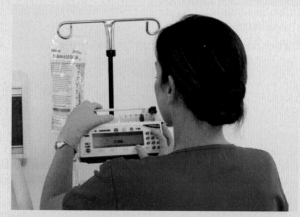

FIGURE 4. Programming mini-infusion pump.

ACTION	RATIONALE
28. Clamp tubing on secondary IV infusion administration set when solution is infused. Follow facility policy regarding disposal of equipment.	Most facilities allow the reuse of tubing, reducing the risk for contamination. The frequency of administration set tubing changes varies.
29. Check rate of primary infusion.	Administration of secondary infusion may interfere with primary infusion rate.
30. Remove PPE, if used. Perform hand hygiene.	Proper removal of PPE reduces the risk for infection transmission and contamination of other items. Hand hygiene prevents the spread of microorganisms.
31. Document the administration of the medication immediately after administration. See Documentation section below. Document the volume of fluid administered on the intake and output record, if necessary.	Timely documentation helps to ensure patient safety.
32. Evaluate the patient's response to the medication within appropriate time frame. Monitor IV site at periodic intervals.	The patient needs to be evaluated for therapeutic and adverse effects from the medication.

EVALUATION

The expected outcomes have been met when the medication has been delivered via the IV route; the patient experiences the intended effect of the medication; the patient experiences no adverse effects; and the patient understands and complies with the medication regimen.

DOCUMENTATION

Guidelines

Document the administration of the medication immediately after administration, including date, time, dose, route of administration, site of administration, and rate of administration on the eMAR/MAR or record using the required format. If using a bar-code system, medication administration is automatically recorded when the bar code is scanned. PRN medications require documentation of the reason for administration. Prompt recording avoids the possibility of accidentally repeating the administration of the drug. If the drug was refused or omitted, record this in the appropriate area on the medication record and notify the primary care provider. This verifies the reason medication was omitted and ensures that health care personnel providing care for the patient are aware of the occurrence. Document the volume of fluid administered on the intake and output record, if necessary.

UNEXPECTED SITUATIONS AND ASSOCIATED INTERVENTIONS

- *Upon assessing the IV site before administering medication, you note that the IV has infiltrated:* Stop IV fluid and remove the IV from the extremity. Restart the IV in a different location. Continue to monitor the new IV site as medication is administered.
- *While administering medication, you note a cloudy, white substance forming in the IV tubing:* Stop the IV from flowing and stop administering the medication to prevent precipitate from entering the patient's circulation. Clamp the IV at the site nearest to the patient. Replace tubing on primary and secondary infusions. Check the literature regarding incompatibilities of medications before administering. Medication infusion may require a second IV site or flushing of tubing before and after administration.
- *While you are administering medication, the patient begins to complain of pain at the IV site:* Stop the medication. Assess the IV site for any signs of complications. Flush the IV with normal saline to check for patency. If the IV site appears within normal limits, resume medication administration at a slower rate and continue to monitor.

(continued)

Skill 12 ▶ Administering an Intermittent Intravenous Infusion of Medication via a Mini-Infusion Pump *(continued)*

SPECIAL CONSIDERATIONS

General Considerations

- Intermittent administration sets disconnected after use should be replaced every 24 hours; repeated disconnection and reconnection increases risk of contamination at the spike end, catheter hub, needleless connector and the end of the administration set, potential increasing the risk for catheter-related bloodstream infection (INS, 2016b)
- Ongoing assessment is an important part of nursing care for both evaluation of patient response to administered medications and early detection of adverse drug reactions. If an adverse effect is suspected, withhold further medication doses and notify the patient's primary care provider. Additional intervention is based on type of reaction and patient assessment.

Infant and Child Considerations

- Infants and small children with fluid restrictions may not tolerate the added IV fluid needed for administration with piggyback systems. The mini-infusion pump should be considered for use with these children.

EVIDENCE FOR PRACTICE ▶

INFUSION NURSING STANDARDS OF PRACTICE

Infusion Nurses Society (INS). (2016b). Infusion therapy. Standards of practice. *Journal of Infusion Nursing, 39*(Suppl 1), S1–S159.

Refer to details in Skill 10, Evidence for Practice.

EVIDENCE FOR PRACTICE ▶

INFUSION NURSING POLICIES AND PROCEDURES FOR INFUSION THERAPY

Infusion Nurses Society (INS). (2016a). *Policies and procedures for infusion therapy* (5th ed.). Norwood, MA: Author.

Refer to details in Skill 10, Evidence for Practice.

Skill 13 ▶ Administering Medications by Intravenous Bolus or Push Through a Medication or Drug-Infusion Lock

A medication or drug-infusion lock, also known as an intermittent peripheral venous access device or saline lock, is used for patients who require intermittent IV medication, but not a continuous IV infusion. This device consists of a catheter connected to a short length of tubing capped with a sealed injection port. After the catheter is in place in the patient's vein, the catheter and tubing are anchored to the patient's arm so that the catheter remains in place until the patient no longer requires the repeated medication intravenously.

The device is kept patent (working) by flushing with small amounts of saline pushed through the device on a routine basis. Using saline eliminates any possible systemic effects on coagulation, development of a heparin allergy, and drug incompatibility, which may occur when a heparin solution is used. The nurse must confirm IV placement before administration of medication. It is important to flush the drug-infusion lock before and after the medication is administered to clear the vein of any medication and to prevent clot formation in the device. If infiltration or phlebitis occurs, the lock is removed and replaced in a new site.

DELEGATION CONSIDERATIONS	The administration of medications through an intermittent peripheral venous access device is not delegated to nursing assistive personnel (NAP) or to unlicensed assistive personnel (UAP). Depending on the state's nurse practice act and the organization's policies and procedures, the administration of specified IV medications in some settings may be delegated to licensed practical/vocational nurses (LPN/LVNs) who have received appropriate training. The decision to delegate must be based on careful analysis of the patient's needs and circumstances, as well as the qualifications of the person to whom the task is being delegated.

EQUIPMENT

- Prescribed medication
- 2 – Normal saline flushes prepared in a syringe (3 to 10 mL) according to facility policy
- Antimicrobial swabs
- Passive disinfection caps (based on facility policy)
- Syringe with a needleless device or 23- to 25-gauge, 1-in needle (follow facility policy)
- Watch or clock with a second hand
- Disposable gloves
- Electronic Medication Administration Record (eMAR) or Medication Administration Record (MAR)
- Additional PPE, as indicated

ASSESSMENT

Assess the appropriateness of the drug for the patient. Review medical history, allergy, assessment, and laboratory data that may influence drug administration. Check the expiration date before administering the medication. Assess the patient's IV site for signs of any complications. Assess the patient's knowledge of the medication. If the patient has a knowledge deficit about the medication, this may be the appropriate time to begin education about the medication. If the medication may affect the patient's vital signs, assess them before administration. If the medication is for pain relief, assess the patient's pain before and after administration. Verify the patient's name, dose, route, and time of administration.

NURSING DIAGNOSIS

Determine related factors for the nursing diagnoses based on the patient's current status. Appropriate nursing diagnoses may include:

- Risk for allergy reaction
- Risk for infection
- Risk for injury

OUTCOME IDENTIFICATION AND PLANNING

The expected outcome to achieve when administering medication via a medication or drug-infusion lock is that the medication is delivered via the IV route and the patient experiences the intended effect of the medication. Other outcomes that may be appropriate include the following: the patient experiences no adverse effects; and the patient understands and complies with the medication regimen.

IMPLEMENTATION

ACTION	RATIONALE
1. Gather equipment. Check the medication order against the original order in the health record, according to facility policy. Clarify any inconsistencies. Check the patient's health record for allergies. Check a drug resource to clarify whether medication needs to be diluted before bolus administration. Verify the recommended administration rate.	This comparison helps to identify errors that may have occurred when orders were transcribed. The primary care provider's order or prescription is the legal record of medication orders for each facility. Recommended administration rate delivers the correct dose of medication as prescribed.
2. Know the actions, special nursing considerations, safe dose ranges, purpose of administration, and adverse effects of the medications to be administered. Consider the appropriateness of the medication for this patient.	This knowledge aids the nurse in evaluating the therapeutic effect of the medication in relation to the patient's disorder and can also be used to educate the patient about the medication.

(continued)

Skill 13 ▶ Administering Medications by Intravenous Bolus or Push Through a Medication or Drug-Infusion Lock *(continued)*

ACTION	RATIONALE

3. Perform hand hygiene.

Hand hygiene prevents the spread of microorganisms.

4. Move the medication supply system to the outside of the patient's room or prepare for administration at the medication supply system in the medication area. Alternatively, access the medication administration supply system at or inside the patient's room.

Organization facilitates error-free administration and saves time.

5. Unlock the medication supply system or drawer. Enter pass code and scan employee identification, if required.

Locking the medication supply system or drawer safeguards each patient's medication supply. Facility accrediting organizations require medication supply systems to be locked when not in use. Entering pass code and scanning ID allows only authorized users into the system and identifies the user for documentation by the computer.

6. **Prepare medication for one patient at a time.**

This prevents errors in medication administration.

7. Read the eMAR/MAR and select the proper medication from medication supply system or the patient's medication drawer.

This is the *first* check of the label.

8. Compare the label with the eMAR/MAR. Check expiration dates and perform calculations, if necessary. Scan the bar code on the package, if required.

This is the *second* check of the label. Verify calculations with another nurse to ensure safety, if necessary.

9. If necessary, withdraw medication from an ampule or vial as described in Skills 3 and 4.

Allows administration of medication.

10. **Depending on facility policy, the third check of the label may occur at this point. If so, when all medications for one patient have been prepared, recheck the labels with the eMAR/MAR before taking the medications to the patient. However, many facilities require the third check to occur at the bedside, after identifying the patient.**

This *third* check ensures accuracy and helps to prevent errors. *Note:* Many facilities require the *third* check to occur at the bedside, after identifying the patient and before administration.

11. **Lock the medication supply system before leaving it.**

Locking the medication supply system or drawer safeguards the patient's medication supply. Facility accrediting organizations require medication supply systems to be locked when not in use.

12. Transport medications and equipment to the patient's bedside carefully, and keep the medications in sight at all times.

Careful handling and close observation prevent accidental or deliberate disarrangement of medications. Having equipment available saves time and facilitates performance of the task.

13. **Ensure that the patient receives the medications at the correct time.**

Check facility policy, which may allow for administration within a period of 30 minutes before or 30 minutes after the designated time.

14. Perform hand hygiene and put on PPE, if indicated.

Hand hygiene and PPE prevent the spread of microorganisms. PPE is required based on transmission precautions.

15. **Identify the patient. Compare the information with the eMAR/MAR. The patient should be identified using at least two of the following methods (The Joint Commission, 2018):**

Identifying the patient ensures the right patient receives the medications and helps prevent errors. The patient's room number or physical location is not used as an identifier (The Joint Commission, 2018). Replace the identification band if it is missing or inaccurate in any way.

ACTION	**RATIONALE**
a. Check the name on the patient's identification band.	This requires a response from the patient, but illness and strange surroundings often cause patients to be confused.
b. Check the identification number on the patient's identification band.	
c. Check the birth date on the patient's identification band.	
d. Ask the patient to state his or her name and birth date, based on facility policy.	
16. Close the door to the room or pull the bedside curtain.	This provides patient privacy.
17. **Complete necessary assessments before administering medications. Check the patient's allergy bracelet or ask the patient about allergies. Explain the purpose and action of the medication to the patient.**	Assessment is a prerequisite to administration of medications. Explanation provides rationale, increases knowledge, and reduces anxiety.
18. Scan the patient's bar code on the identification band, if required (Figure 1).	Scanning provides an additional check to ensure that the medication is given to the right patient.
19. **Based on facility policy, the third check of the label may occur at this point. If so, recheck the labels with the eMAR/MAR before administering the medications to the patient.**	Many facilities require the *third* check to occur at the bedside, after identifying the patient and before administration. If facility policy directs the *third* check at this time, this *third* check ensures accuracy and helps to prevent errors.
20. Assess IV site for presence of inflammation or infiltration.	IV medication must be given directly into a vein for safe administration.
21. Put on clean gloves.	Gloves protect the nurse's hands from contact with the patient's blood.
22. Remove the passive disinfection cap from the needleless connector or access port of the medication lock (Figure 2). Alternatively, if a passive disinfection cap is not in place, use an antimicrobial swab to vigorously scrub the needleless connector or access port of the medication lock and allow to dry.	Passive disinfection caps contain an antiseptic-impregnated sponge that dispenses the antiseptic over the connector's top and threads, and protects the hub from contamination by touch or airborne sources (Stango et al., 2014). Venous access device entry points, end-caps, and needleless connectors must be vigorously scrubbed and disinfected prior to each access to reduce the risk for introduction of microorganisms and prevent venous access device-related infection (Frimpong et al., 2015; Harper, 2014; INS, 2016b; The Joint Commission, 2018; Loveday, 2014). Friction is needed to physically remove microorganisms from the top, sides, and threads of the needleless connector or end cap. Allow the antiseptic to dry completely (15 to 30 seconds) to ensure complete effectiveness (Harper).

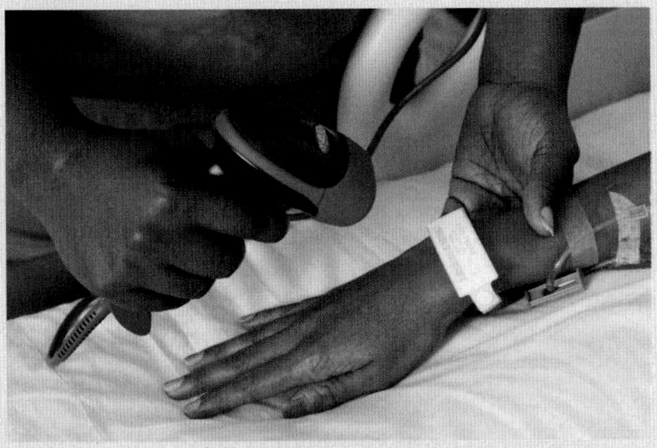

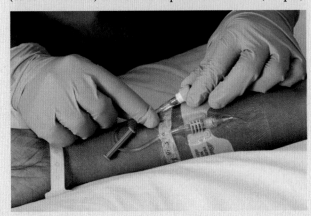

FIGURE 1. Scanning bar code on patient's identification bracelet.

FIGURE 2. Removing the passive disinfection cap from the access port.

(continued)

Skill 13 Administering Medications by Intravenous Bolus or Push Through a Medication or Drug-Infusion Lock *(continued)*

ACTION

23. Uncap saline flush syringe. Stabilize the port with your nondominant hand and insert the saline flush syringe into the needleless connector or end cap on the access port of the medication lock (Figure 3).

24. Release the clamp on the extension tubing of the medication lock (Figure 4). Pull back on the syringe plunger to aspirate the catheter for positive blood return (Figure 5). If positive, instill the solution over 1 minute or flush the line according to facility policy. Observe the insertion site while inserting the saline. Remove syringe.

RATIONALE

Assessing patency of venous access device is necessary to ensure intravenous administration of the medication.

Positive blood return confirms patency before administration of medications and solutions (INS, 2016b). Flushing without incident ensures patency of the IV line and administration of medication into the bloodstream. Puffiness, pain, or swelling as the site is flushed could indicate infiltration of the catheter.

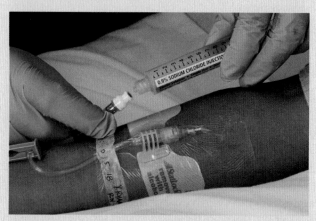

FIGURE 3. Inserting the saline flush syringe into the access port.

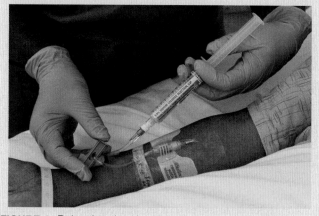

FIGURE 4. Releasing the clamp on the extension tubing.

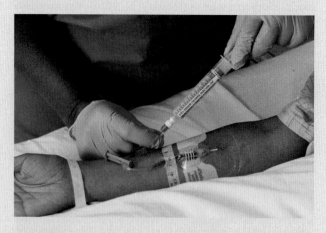

FIGURE 5. Pulling back on the plunger to aspirate for a blood return.

25. Use an antimicrobial swab to vigorously scrub the needleless connector or end cap on the access port of the medication lock and allow to dry.

Venous access device entry points, end-caps, and needleless connectors must be vigorously scrubbed and disinfected prior to each access to reduce the risk for introduction of microorganisms and prevent venous access device-related infection (Frimpong et al., 2015; Harper, 2014; INS, 2016b; The Joint Commission, 2018; Loveday, 2014). Friction is needed to physically remove microorganisms from the top, sides, and threads of the needleless connector or end cap. Allow the antiseptic to dry completely (15 to 30 seconds) to ensure complete effectiveness (Harper).

ACTION	RATIONALE
26. Uncap the medication syringe. Insert the medication syringe into the needleless connector or end cap on the access port of the medication lock. Using a watch or clock with a second-hand to time the rate, **inject the medication at the recommended rate (Figure 6). Do not force the injection if resistance is felt.**	This delivers the correct amount of medication at the proper interval. Easy installation of medication usually indicates that the lock is still patent and in the vein. If force is used against resistance, a clot may break away and cause a blockage elsewhere in the body.
27. While administering the medication, observe the infusion site and assess patient for any adverse reaction. If signs of adverse reaction occur, stop infusion immediately and notify the primary health provider.	Signs of adverse reaction, such as peripheral IV infiltration, rash or itching, or pain at the infusion, necessitate stopping of administration of the drug (INS, 2016a).
28. Remove the medication syringe from the access port. Use a new antimicrobial swab to vigorously scrub the needleless connector or end cap on the access port and allow to dry. Stabilize the port with your nondominant hand. Uncap the second saline flush syringe. Insert the saline flush syringe into the needleless connector or end cap on the access port. Instill the flush solution at the same rate as the administered medication (INS, 2016a).	Venous access device entry points, end-caps, and needleless connectors must be vigorously scrubbed and disinfected prior to each access to reduce the risk for introduction of microorganisms and prevent venous access device-related infection (Frimpong et al., 2015; Harper, 2014; INS, 2016b; The Joint Commission, 2018; Loveday, 2014). Friction is needed to physically remove microorganisms from the top, sides, and threads of the needleless connector or end cap. Allow the antiseptic to dry completely (15 to 30 seconds) to ensure complete effectiveness (Harper). Flushing after medication administration ensure the entire drug dose has been cleared from the extension tubing on the venous access device or from the infusion system and prevents precipitation due to solution/medication incompatibility (INS, 2016a).
29. If the medication lock is capped with positive pressure valve/device, remove syringe, and then clamp the extension tubing (Figure 7). Alternatively, to gain positive pressure if positive pressure valve/device is not present, clamp the extension tubing as you are still flushing the last of the saline into the medication lock. Remove syringe.	Positive pressure prevents blood from backing into the catheter and causing the medication lock to clot off.

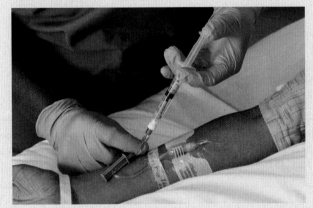

FIGURE 6. Injecting the medication at the recommended rate.

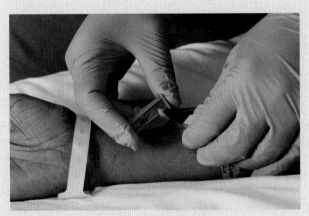

FIGURE 7. Clamping the extension tubing.

(continued)

Skill 13 ▶ Administering Medications by Intravenous Bolus or Push Through a Medication or Drug-Infusion Lock *(continued)*

ACTION	RATIONALE
30. Using an antimicrobial swab, vigorously scrub the needleless connector or end cap on the access port of the medication lock and allow to dry. Attach a passive disinfection cap to the needleless connector or end cap on the access port of the medication lock (Figure 8).	Venous access device entry points, end-caps, and needleless connectors must be vigorously scrubbed and disinfected prior to each access to reduce the risk for introduction of microorganisms and prevent venous access device-related infection (Frimpong et al., 2015; Harper, 2014; INS, 2016b; The Joint Commission, 2018; Loveday et al., 2014). Friction is needed to physically remove microorganisms from the top, sides, and threads of the needleless connector or end cap. Allow the antiseptic to dry completely (15 to 30 seconds) to ensure complete effectiveness (Harper, 2014). Passive disinfection caps contain an antiseptic-impregnated sponge that dispenses the antiseptic over the connector's top and threads, and protect the hub from contamination by touch or airborne sources (Stango et al., 2014).

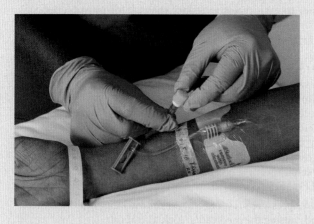

FIGURE 8. Attaching a passive disinfection cap to the access port.

31. Discard the syringe in the appropriate receptacle.	Proper disposal prevents injury and the spread of microorganisms.
32. Remove gloves and additional PPE, if used. Perform hand hygiene.	Proper removal of PPE reduces the risk for infection transmission and contamination of other items. Hand hygiene prevents the spread of microorganisms.
33. Document the administration of the medication immediately after administration. See Documentation section below.	Timely documentation helps to ensure patient safety.
34. Evaluate the patient's response to the medication within an appropriate time frame.	The patient needs to be evaluated for therapeutic and adverse effects from the medication.

EVALUATION   The expected outcomes have been met when the medication is delivered via the IV route; the patient experiences the intended effect of the medication; the patient experiences no adverse effects; and the patient understands and complies with the medication regimen.

DOCUMENTATION

Guidelines   Document the administration of the medication and saline flush, including date, time, dose, route of administration, site of administration, and rate of administration on the eMAR/MAR or record using the required format, immediately after administration. If using a bar-code system, medication administration is automatically recorded when the bar code is scanned. PRN medications require documentation of the reason for administration. Prompt recording avoids the possibility of accidentally repeating the administration of the drug. If the drug was refused or omitted, record this in the appropriate area on the medication record and notify the primary care provider. This verifies the reason medication was omitted and ensures that the health care personnel providing care for the patient are aware of the occurrence.

UNEXPECTED SITUATIONS AND ASSOCIATED INTERVENTIONS	• *Upon assessing the medication lock site before administering the medication, you note that the medication lock has infiltrated:* Remove the medication lock from the extremity. Restart peripheral venous access in a different location. Continue to monitor the new site as medication is administered. • *While you are administering medication, the patient begins to complain of pain at the site:* Stop the medication. Assess the medication lock site for signs of infiltration and phlebitis. Flush the medication lock with normal saline again to recheck patency. If the IV site appears within normal limits, resume medication administration at a slower rate. If pain persists, stop, remove medication lock and restart in a different location. • *As you are attempting to access the lock, the syringe tip touches the patient's arm:* Discard syringe. Prepare a new dose for administration. • *No blood return is noted upon aspiration:* If the medication lock appears patent, without signs of infiltration, and normal saline fluid infuses without difficulty, proceed with administration. Observe closely for signs and symptoms of infiltration during and after administration.
SPECIAL CONSIDERATIONS *General Considerations*	• Vascular access devices should also be "locked" after completion of the flush solution at each use to decrease the risk of occlusion and catheter-related bloodstream infection (INS, 2016b). According to the guidelines from the INS (2016b), short peripheral catheters are locked with normal saline solution. If the device is not in use, periodic flushing according to facility policy is required to keep the catheter patent. • Previously, recommendations suggested routine rotation of insertions sites at various intervals, usually 72 to 96 hours. Current research and guidelines support maintaining peripheral IV access devices until no longer clinically indicated or until a complication develops (Bolton, 2015; INS, 2016a; Loveday et al., 2014; Tuffaha et al., 2014). Nurses should use clinical assessment and judgment in deciding when to replace or discontinue a peripheral IV catheter. • The clinical need for the IV catheter should be assessed on a daily basis (INS, 2016a). Assessment is based on the patient's overall condition, access site, skin and wound integrity, length and type of therapy, and the integrity of the device, dressing and stabilization device (Helton et al., 2016). The device insertion site and dressing should be assessed every 4 hours at a minimum (INS, 2016a). • Ongoing assessment is an important part of nursing care to evaluate patient response to administered medications and early detection of adverse reactions. If an adverse effect is suspected, withhold further medication doses and notify the patient's primary health care provider. Additional intervention is based on type of reaction and patient assessment.
Infant and Child Considerations	• If the volume of medication being administered is small (less than 1.0 mL), always include the amount of flush solution as part of the total amount to be injected and take this into account when determining how fast to push a medication. For example, if the medication is to be injected at a rate of 1.0 mL per minute and the total amount of solution to be injected is 2.25 mL (0.25-mL medication volume plus 2.0-mL saline flush solution volume equals 2.25 mL), then the medication would be injected over a period of 2 minutes 15 seconds.

(continued)

Skill 13 ▶ Administering Medications by Intravenous Bolus or Push Through a Medication or Drug-Infusion Lock *(continued)*

EVIDENCE FOR PRACTICE ▶	**INFUSION NURSING STANDARDS OF PRACTICE** Infusion Nurses Society (INS). (2016b). Infusion therapy. Standards of practice. *Journal of Infusion Nursing, 39*(Suppl 1), S1–S159. Refer to details in Skill 10, Evidence for Practice.

EVIDENCE FOR PRACTICE ▶	**INFUSION NURSING POLICIES AND PROCEDURES FOR INFUSION THERAPY** Infusion Nurses Society (INS). (2016a). *Policies and procedures for infusion therapy* (5th ed.). Norwood, MA: Author. Refer to details in Skill 10, Evidence for Practice.

Skill 14 ▶ Administering Medication via a Metered-Dose Inhaler (MDI)

Drugs for **inhalation** may be administered via a **metered-dose inhaler** (MDI). An MDI is a handheld inhaler that uses an aerosol spray or mist to deliver a controlled dose of medication with each compression of the canister that is then breathed in by the patient. The medication is then absorbed rapidly through the lung tissue, resulting in local and systemic effects. There are two methods for using an MDI; the preferred method is with a device called a valved holding chamber or spacer, and is outlined in the steps in the following skill (Cleveland Clinic, 2014). An MDI can also be used without a chamber. Refer to the accompanying Skill Variation at the end of this skill. Patients should discuss which method is most appropriate for use with their health care provider. There are a number of different medication inhaler devices. It is imperative that nurses understand the administration technique for the specific type of inhaler in use in order to administer the prescribed medication effectively and to provide appropriate patient education (Alismail et al., 2016).

DELEGATION CONSIDERATIONS

The administration of medication via a metered-dose inhaler is not delegated to nursing assistive personnel (NAP) or to unlicensed assistive personnel (UAP). Depending on the state's nurse practice act and the organization's policies and procedures, administration of a metered-dose inhaler may be delegated to licensed practical/vocational nurses (LPN/LVNs). The decision to delegate must be based on careful analysis of the patient's needs and circumstances, as well as the qualifications of the person to whom the task is being delegated.

EQUIPMENT

- Stethoscope
- Medication in an MDI
- Spacer or holding chamber
- Electronic Medication Administration Record (eMAR) or Medication Administration Record (MAR)
- PPE, as indicated

ASSESSMENT   Assess the appropriateness of the drug for the patient. Review medical history, allergy, assessment, and laboratory data that may influence drug administration. Assess respiratory rate, rhythm, and depth to establish a baseline. Assess lung sounds before and after use to establish a baseline and determine the effectiveness of the medication. If appropriate and/or ordered, assess oxygen saturation level before medication administration. The oxygenation level usually increases after the medication is administered. Assess the patient's ability to manage an MDI; young and older adults may have dexterity problems. Assess the patient's knowledge and understanding of the medication's purpose and action. Verify patient name, dose, route, and time of administration.

NURSING DIAGNOSIS   Determine related factors for the nursing diagnoses based on the patient's current status. Appropriate nursing diagnoses may include:

- Risk for activity intolerance
- Impaired gas exchange
- Deficient knowledge

OUTCOME IDENTIFICATION AND PLANNING   The expected outcome to achieve when using an MDI is that the medication is administered and breathed in by the patient and the patient experiences the intended effect of the medication. Other outcomes that may be appropriate include the following: the patient understands the rationale for the inhaled medication; and the patient demonstrates correct use of an MDI.

IMPLEMENTATION

ACTION	RATIONALE
1. Gather equipment. Check each medication order against the original order in the health record, according to facility policy. Clarify any inconsistencies. Check the patient's health record for allergies.	This comparison helps to identify errors that may have occurred when orders were transcribed. The primary care provider's order or prescription is the legal record of medication orders for each facility.
2. Know the actions, special nursing considerations, safe dose ranges, purpose of administration, and adverse effects of the medications to be administered. Consider the appropriateness of the medication for this patient.	This knowledge aids the nurse in evaluating the therapeutic effect of the medication in relation to the patient's disorder and can also be used to educate the patient about the medication.
3. Perform hand hygiene.	Hand hygiene prevents the spread of microorganisms.
4. Move the medication supply system to the outside of the patient's room or prepare for administration at the medication supply system in the medication area. Alternatively, access the medication administration supply system at or inside the patient's room.	Organization facilitates error-free administration and saves time.
5. Unlock the medication supply system or drawer. Enter pass code and scan employee identification, if required.	Locking the medication supply system or drawer safeguards each patient's medication supply. Facility accrediting organizations require medication supply systems to be locked when not in use. Entering pass code and scanning ID allows only authorized users into the computer system and identifies the user for documentation by the computer.
6. **Prepare medications for one patient at a time.**	This prevents errors in medication administration.
7. Read the eMAR/MAR and select the proper medication from the patient's medication drawer or medication supply system.	This is the *first* check of the label.
8. Compare the label with the eMAR/MAR. Check expiration dates and perform calculations, if necessary. Scan the bar code on the package, if required.	This is the *second* check of the label. Verify calculations with another nurse to ensure safety, if necessary.

(continued)

Skill 14 ▶ Administering Medication via a Metered-Dose Inhaler (MDI) *(continued)*

ACTION	RATIONALE
9. Depending on facility policy, the third check of the label may occur at this point. If so, when all medications for one patient have been prepared, recheck the labels with the eMAR/MAR before taking the medications to the patient. However, many facilities require the third check to occur at the bedside, after identifying the patient.	This *third* check ensures accuracy and helps to prevent errors. *Note:* Many facilities require the *third* check to occur at the bedside, after identifying the patient and before administration.
10. Lock the medication supply system before leaving it.	Locking the medication supply system or drawer safeguards the patient's medication supply. Facility accrediting organizations require medication supply systems to be locked when not in use.
11. Transport medications to the patient's bedside carefully, and keep the medications in sight at all times.	Careful handling and close observation prevent accidental or deliberate disarrangement of medications.
12. Ensure that the patient receives the medications at the correct time.	Check facility policy, which may allow for administration within a period of 30 minutes before or 30 minutes after the designated time.
13. Perform hand hygiene and put on PPE, if indicated.	Hand hygiene and PPE prevent the spread of microorganisms. PPE is required based on transmission precautions.
14. Identify the patient. Compare the information with the eMAR/MAR. The patient should be identified using at least two of the following methods (The Joint Commission, 2018):	Identifying the patient ensures the right patient receives the medications and helps prevent errors. The patient's room number or physical location is not used as an identifier (The Joint Commission, 2018). Replace the identification band if it is missing or inaccurate in any way.
a. Check the name on the patient's identification band.	This requires a response from the patient, but illness and strange surroundings often cause patients to be confused.
b. Check the identification number on the patient's identification band.	
c. Check the birth date on the patient's identification band.	
d. Ask the patient to state his or her name and birth date, based on facility policy.	
15. Complete necessary assessments before administering medications. Check the patient's allergy bracelet or ask the patient about allergies. Explain what you are going to do and the reason for doing it to the patient.	Assessment is a prerequisite to administration of medications. Explanation relieves anxiety and facilitates cooperation.
16. Scan the patient's bar code on the identification band, if required (Figure 1).	Provides an additional check to ensure that the medication is given to the right patient.

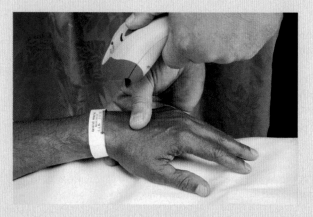

FIGURE 1. Scanning bar code on patient's identification bracelet.

ACTION	RATIONALE

ACTION

17. **Based on facility policy, the third check of the label may occur at this point. If so, recheck the labels with the eMAR/MAR before administering the medications to the patient.**

18. Shake the inhaler well.

19. Remove the mouthpiece cover from the MDI and the spacer. Attach the MDI to the spacer by inserting in the open end of the spacer, opposite the mouthpiece. (Refer to the accompanying Skill Variation for using an MDI without a spacer.)

20. Have patient place the spacer's mouthpiece into mouth, grasping securely with teeth and sealing the lips tightly around the mouthpiece (Figure 2). Have patient breathe normally through the spacer.

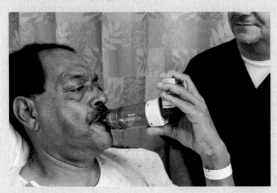

RATIONALE

Many facilities require the *third* check to occur at the bedside, after identifying the patient and before administration. If facility policy directs the *third* check at this time, this *third* check ensures accuracy and helps to prevent errors.

The medication and propellant may separate when the canister is not in use. Shaking well ensures that the patient is receiving the correct dosage of medication.

The use of a spacer or valved holding chamber is preferred because it traps the medication and aids in delivery of the correct dose.

Medication should not leak out around the mouthpiece.

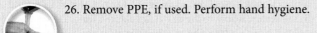
FIGURE 2. Placing spacer with MDI into mouth.

21. The patient should breathe out completely, then depress the canister once, releasing one puff into the spacer, then inhale slowly and deeply through the mouth.

22. **Instruct patient to hold his or her breath for 5 to 10 seconds, or as long as possible, and then to exhale slowly through pursed lips.**

23. Wait 1 to 5 minutes, as prescribed, before administering the next puff, as prescribed.

24. After the prescribed number of puffs has been administered, have the patient remove the MDI from the spacer and replace the caps on both MDI and spacer.

25. Have the patient gargle and rinse with tap water after using an MDI, as necessary. Clean the MDI according to the manufacturer's directions.

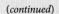 26. Remove PPE, if used. Perform hand hygiene.

The spacer will hold the medication in suspension for a short period so that the patient can receive more of the prescribed medication than if it had been projected into the air. Breathing slowly and deeply distributes the medication deep into the airways.

This allows better distribution of the medication to the airways and longer absorption time for the medication.

This ensures that both puffs are absorbed as much as possible. Bronchodilation after the first puff allows for deeper penetration by subsequent puffs.

By replacing the caps, the patient is preventing any dust or dirt from entering and being propelled into the bronchioles with later doses.

Rinsing removes medication residue from the mouth. Rinsing is necessary when using inhaled steroids because oral fungal infections can occur. The buildup of medication in the device can attract bacteria and affect how the medication is delivered.

Proper removal of PPE reduces the risk for infection transmission and contamination of other items. Hand hygiene prevents the spread of microorganisms.

(continued)

Skill 14 ▶ **Administering Medication via a Metered-Dose Inhaler (MDI)** *(continued)*

ACTION	RATIONALE
27. Document the administration of the medication immediately after administration. See Documentation section below.	Timely documentation helps to ensure patient safety.
28. Evaluate the patient's response to the medication within an appropriate time frame. Reassess lung sounds, oxygen saturation level, and respirations, as indicated.	The patient needs to be evaluated for therapeutic and adverse effects from the medication.

EVALUATION

The expected outcomes have been met when the medication is administered and breathed in by the patient; the patient experiences the intended effect of the medication; the patient understands the rationale for the inhaled medication; and the patient demonstrated correct use of the MDI.

DOCUMENTATION

Guidelines

Document the administration of the medication immediately after administration, including date, time, dose, route of administration and any teaching done with the patient on the eMAR/MAR or record using the required format. If using a bar-code system, medication administration is recorded automatically when the bar code is scanned. PRN medications require documentation of the reason for administration. Prompt recording avoids the possibility of accidentally repeating the administration of the drug. Document respiratory rate, oxygen saturation, if applicable, lung assessment, and the patient's response to the treatment, if appropriate. If the drug was refused or omitted, record this in the appropriate area on the medication record and notify the primary care provider. This verifies the reason medication was omitted and ensures that health care personnel providing care for the patient are aware of the occurrence.

Sample Documentation

> 9/29/20 0820 Wheezes noted in all lobes of lungs before albuterol MDI, O_2 saturation 92%, respiratory rate 24 breaths per minute. After albuterol treatment, lung sounds are clear and equal in all lobes, O_2 saturation 97%, respiratory rate 18 breaths per minute. Patient able to demonstrate accurately the use of an MDI and spacer and verbalizes understanding of medication purpose and action.
>
> —*C. Bausler, RN*

UNEXPECTED SITUATIONS AND ASSOCIATED INTERVENTIONS

- *Patient uses MDI, but symptoms are not relieved:* Check to make sure that the inhaler still contains medication. The patient may have received only propellant, without medication.
- *Patient is unable to use MDI:* Many companies have adaptive devices that allow patients to use MDIs.
- *Patient reports that relief of symptoms has decreased, even with increased number of puffs:* Have patient demonstrate the technique that he or she is using. Many patients lack an understanding of correct use of an MDI and/or develop poor habits over time (Levy, Hardwell, McKnight, & Holmes., 2013). Poor administration technique can lead to a decrease in effectiveness and a need for an increased dosage of medication.

SPECIAL CONSIDERATIONS

General Considerations

- The plastic holder and provided with the inhaler should be cleaned at least weekly. Remove the medication canister and clean with warm running water. Shake the holder and allow to air dry.
- Some medication canisters cannot be removed from the plastic holder. Wipe the mouthpiece with a cloth or dry cotton swab and/or refer to the manufacturer's directions for cleaning (Cleveland Clinic, 2014).
- Clean the spacer (valved holding chamber) once a week by soaking in warm water with a mild detergent. Rinse well and shake off excess water. Allow to air dry (Cleveland Clinic, 2014).
- Do not store spacer (valved holding chamber) in a plastic bag to prevent moisture retention and possible resulting microorganism growth.

- If the medication being administered is a steroid, the patient should rinse the mouth with water after administration to prevent irritation and secondary infection to the oral mucosa (Cleveland Clinic, 2014).
- Ongoing assessment is an important part of nursing care to evaluate patient response to administered medications and early detection of adverse reactions. If an adverse effect is suspected, withhold further medication doses and notify the patient's primary care provider. Additional intervention is based on type of reaction and patient assessment.

Infant and Child Considerations

- Young children usually require a spacer to use an MDI. Spacers with masks are available for young children; consider using these for children under 5 years of age to aid in the delivery of the medication. The mask must fit securely over both the nose and the mouth to ensure a good seal and prevent medication from escaping.
- Children must be able to seal their lips around the mouthpiece in order to use a spacer without a mask.
- Many medications can also be administered as a nebulizer (see Skill 16).

Home Care Considerations

- It is important for patients to know how to tell when medication levels are getting low. The most reliable method is to look on the canister and see how many puffs the canister contains. Divide this number by the number of puffs used daily to ascertain how many days the MDI will last. For instance, if the MDI contains 200 puffs and the patient takes 6 puffs per day, the MDI should last for 33 days. Keep a diary or record of inhaler use and discard the inhaler on reaching the labeled number of doses. This method may be cumbersome and impractical for some patients, but it is a reliable way to determine how much medication remains in an MDI. Another accurate way to know when the canister is depleted is to use a dose counter, which counts down each time the canister is activated (Cleveland Clinic, 2014). **Floating the canister in water is not reliable and is contraindicated. Immersion in water can cause valve obstruction and threatens product integrity (MedlinePlus, 2016b; Rubin, 2010).**

Skill Variation ▶ Using an MDI Without a Spacer

Prepare medication as outlined in steps 1–17 above (Skill 14).

1. Remove the cap from the MDI. Shake the inhaler well.
2. Have the patient take a deep breath and exhale.
3. Have the patient hold the inhaler 1 to 2 in away from the mouth (about the width of 2 fingers [MedlinePlus, 2016b]) (Figure A). Have the patient begin to inhale slowly and deeply, depress the medication canister, and continue to inhale for a full breath.
4. **Instruct the patient to hold the breath for 5 to 10 seconds, or as long as possible, and then to exhale slowly through pursed lips.**
5. **Wait 1 to 5 minutes, as prescribed, before administering the next puff.**
6. After the prescribed number of puffs has been administered, have the patient replace the cap on the MDI.
7. Remove additional PPE, if used. Perform hand hygiene.
8. Document administration of the medication on the eMAR/MAR immediately after administering the medication.
9. Evaluate the patient's response to the medication within an appropriate time frame. Reassess lung sounds, oxygen saturation level, if ordered, and respirations.

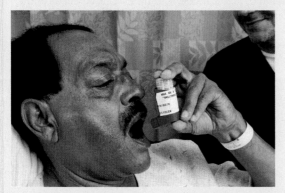

FIGURE A. Holding the MDI 1 to 2 in from the mouth.

(continued)

Skill 14 ▶ Administering Medication via a Metered-Dose Inhaler (MDI) *(continued)*

EVIDENCE FOR PRACTICE ▶

INHALED MEDICATIONS

Correct use of a metered-dose inhaler is critical to ensure accurate dosing of medication. Patients who are prescribed medications delivered with an MDI must have accurate knowledge and demonstrate appropriate technique regarding use to ensure accurate medication delivery. Nurses play a key role in patient education and must have adequate knowledge to provide appropriate educational intervention.

Related Research

De Tratto, K., Gomez, C., Ryan, C. J., Bracken, N., Steffen, A., & Corbridge, S. J. (2014). Nurses' knowledge of inhaler technique in the inpatient hospital setting. *Clinical Nurse Specialist: The Journal for Advanced Nursing Practice, 28* (3), 156–160.

The purpose of this study was to examine inpatient staff nurses' self-perceptions of their inhaler technique knowledge, frequency of providing patient education and responsibility for providing education. The study also assessed the nurses demonstrated inhaler technique using both a metered-dose inhaler (MDI) and diskus (a dry powder inhaler). A total of 100 nurses at a large urban academic medical center working on inpatient medical units agreed to participate. Participants completed a Likert-scale written survey to measure self-perceptions of inhaler technique and frequency and responsibility of patient education regarding MDI and diskus inhaler discharge teaching. Participating nurses then demonstrated inhaler-use technique to a data collector who utilized a detailed, validated checklist outlining the steps for use of both types of inhalers to evaluate the nurses' performance. Misuse of both MDI and diskus technique was defined for the study as having less than 75% of the steps correct (<9 of 12 steps for MDI and <8 steps for diskus). Overall misuse rates for both MDI (82%) and diskus (92%) devices were high, with poor correlation between perceived ability and investigator-measured level of performance of inhaler technique. Key steps missed in use of the devices included breathing out fully prior to inhaling with both devices. Ninety percent of participants missed keeping the device horizontal and 78% did not breathe in quickly during use of the diskus. Frequency of teaching for the diskus device by nurses was correlated with higher scores on the validated checklist, but this was not the case with the MDI. The researchers concluded that although nurses are a key component of patient education, nursing staff lack adequate knowledge of inhaler technique.

Relevance to Nursing Practice

Nurses play a large role in patient education and in designing interventions to positively impact patient outcomes. Accurate dosing of inhaled medications, and therefore control of symptoms and disease treatment, depends on correct use of the delivery device. Providing patient education related to self-administration of medications, leading to accurate medication dosing, is a very important nursing intervention. Nurses must take responsibility for acquiring and maintaining accurate knowledge with regard to use of these devices in order to provide accurate patient teaching. Nurses may advocate for education regarding inhaler technique as part of facility-wide professional development interventions.

Skill 15 ▶ Administering Medication via a Dry Powder Inhaler

Drugs for inhalation may be administered via a dry powder inhaler (DPI). A DPI is a handheld inhaler (diskus) that uses a dry powder form of medication, either in a small capsule or disk inserted into the DPI, or in a compartment inside the DPI. DPIs are breath activated. A quick breath by the patient activates the flow of medication, eliminating the need to coordinate activating the inhaler (spraying the medicine) while inhaling the medicine. However, the drug output and size distribution of the aerosol from a DPI is more or less dependent on the flow rate through the device, so the patient must be able to take a powerful, deep inspiration (Alismail et al., 2016). The medication is then absorbed rapidly through the lung tissue, resulting in local and systemic effects.

Many types of DPIs are available, with distinctive operating instructions. Some have to be loaded with a dose of medication each time they are used and some hold a number of preloaded doses. It is important to understand the particular instructions both for the medication and for the particular delivery device being used.

DELEGATION CONSIDERATIONS	The administration of medication via a dry powder inhaler is not delegated to nursing assistive personnel (NAP) or to unlicensed assistive personnel (UAP). Depending on the state's nurse practice act and the organization's policies and procedures, administration of medication using a dry powder inhaler may be delegated to licensed practical/vocational nurses (LPN/LVNs). The decision to delegate must be based on careful analysis of the patient's needs and circumstances, as well as the qualifications of the person to whom the task is being delegated.
EQUIPMENT	• Stethoscope • DPI and appropriate medication • Electronic Medication Administration Record (eMAR) or Medication Administration Record (MAR) • PPE, as indicated
ASSESSMENT	Assess the appropriateness of the drug for the patient. Review medical history, allergy, assessment, and laboratory data that may influence drug administration. Assess respiratory rate, rhythm, and depth to establish a baseline. Assess lung sounds before and after use to establish a baseline and determine the effectiveness of the medication. If appropriate and/or ordered, assess oxygen saturation level before medication administration. The oxygenation level usually increases after the medication is administered. Assess the patient's ability to manage a DPI. Assess the patient's knowledge and understanding of the medication's purpose and action. Verify patient name, dose, route, and time of administration.
NURSING DIAGNOSIS	Determine related factors for the nursing diagnoses based on the patient's current status. Appropriate nursing diagnoses may include: • Deficient knowledge • Risk for activity intolerance • Impaired gas exchange
OUTCOME IDENTIFICATION AND PLANNING	The expected outcome to achieve is that the medication is administered and breathed in by the patient and the patient experiences the intended effect of the medication. Other outcomes that may be appropriate include the following: the patient understands the rationale for the inhaled medication; and the patient demonstrates correct use of the DPI.

(continued)

Skill 15 ▶ Administering Medication via a Dry Powder Inhaler *(continued)*

IMPLEMENTATION

ACTION	RATIONALE

1. Gather equipment. Check each medication order against the original order in the health record, according to facility policy. Clarify any inconsistencies. Check the patient's health record for allergies.

   This comparison helps to identify errors that may have occurred when orders were transcribed. The primary care provider's order or prescription is the legal record of medication orders for each facility.

2. Know the actions, special nursing considerations, safe dose ranges, purpose of administration, and adverse effects of the medications to be administered. Consider the appropriateness of the medication for this patient.

   This knowledge aids the nurse in evaluating the therapeutic effect of the medication in relation to the patient's disorder and can also be used to educate the patient about the medication.

3. Perform hand hygiene.

   Hand hygiene prevents the spread of microorganisms.

4. Move the medication supply system to the outside of the patient's room or prepare for administration at the medication supply system in the medication area. Alternatively, access the medication administration supply system at or inside the patient's room.

   Organization facilitates error-free administration and saves time.

5. Unlock the medication supply system or drawer. Enter pass code and scan employee identification, if required.

   Locking the medication supply system or drawer safeguards each patient's medication supply. Facility accrediting organizations require medication supply systems to be locked when not in use. Entering pass code and scanning ID allows only authorized users into the system and identifies the user for documentation by the computer.

6. **Prepare medications for one patient at a time.**

   This prevents errors in medication administration.

7. Read the eMAR/MAR and select the proper medication from the patient's medication drawer or medication supply system.

   This is the *first* check of the label.

8. Compare the label with the eMAR/MAR. Check expiration dates and perform calculations, if necessary. Scan the bar code on the package, if required.

   This is the *second* check of the label. Verify calculations with another nurse to ensure safety, if necessary.

9. **Depending on facility policy, the third check of the label may occur at this point. If so, when all medications for one patient have been prepared, recheck the labels with the eMAR/MAR before taking the medications to the patient. However, many facilities require the third check to occur at the bedside, after identifying the patient.**

   This *third* check ensures accuracy and helps to prevent errors. *Note:* Many facilities require the *third* check to occur at the bedside, after identifying the patient and before administration.

10. **Lock the medication supply system before leaving it.**

    Locking the medication supply system or drawer safeguards the patient's medication supply. Facility accrediting organizations require medication supply systems to be locked when not in use.

11. Transport medications to the patient's bedside carefully, and keep the medications in sight at all times.

    Careful handling and close observation prevent accidental or deliberate disarrangement of medications.

12. **Ensure that the patient receives the medications at the correct time.**

    Check facility policy, which may allow for administration within a period of 30 minutes before or 30 minutes after the designated time.

13. Perform hand hygiene and put on PPE, if indicated.

    Hand hygiene and PPE prevent the spread of microorganisms. PPE is required based on transmission precautions.

ACTION	RATIONALE

14. **Identify the patient. Compare the information with the eMAR/MAR. The patient should be identified using at least two of the following methods (The Joint Commission, 2018):**

Identifying the patient ensures the right patient receives the medications and helps prevent errors. The patient's room number or physical location is not used as an identifier (The Joint Commission, 2018). Replace the identification band if it is missing or inaccurate in any way.

a. Check the name on the patient's identification band.

b. Check the identification number on the patient's identification band.

c. Check the birth date on the patient's identification band.

d. Ask the patient to state his or her name and birth date, based on facility policy.

This requires a response from the patient, but illness and strange surroundings often cause patients to be confused.

15. **Complete necessary assessments before administering medications. Check the patient's allergy bracelet or ask the patient about allergies. Explain what you are going to do, and the reason for doing it, to the patient.**

Assessment is a prerequisite to administration of medications.

16. Scan the patient's bar code on the identification band, if required (Figure 1).

Provides an additional check to ensure that the medication is given to the right patient.

17. **Based on facility policy, the third check of the label may occur at this point. If so, recheck the labels with the eMAR/MAR before administering the medications to the patient.**

Many facilities require the *third* check to occur at the bedside, after identifying the patient and before administration. If facility policy directs the *third* check at this time, this *third* check ensures accuracy and helps to prevent errors.

18. Remove the mouthpiece cover or remove the device from storage container. Load a dose into the device as directed by the manufacturer, if necessary. Alternatively, activate the inhaler, if necessary, according to manufacturer's directions.

This is necessary to deliver the medication.

19. Have the patient breathe out slowly and completely, without breathing into the DPI.

This allows for deeper inhalation with the medication dose. Moisture from the patient's breath can clog the inhaler.

20. Instruct the patient to place teeth over, and seal lips around, the mouthpiece. **It is important to not block the opening with the tongue or teeth** (Figure 2).

Prevents medication from escaping and allows for a tight seal, ensuring maximal dosing of medication. Blocking of opening interferes with medication delivery.

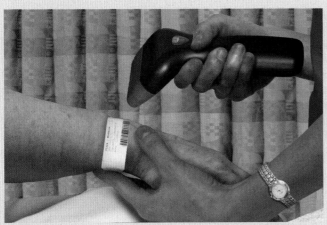

FIGURE 1. Scanning bar code on patient's identification bracelet. (*Photo by B. Proud.*)

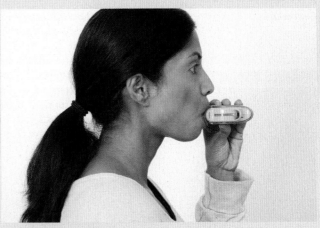

FIGURE 2. Patient with teeth over and lips sealed around mouthpiece.

(*continued*)

Skill 15 ▶ Administering Medication via a Dry Powder Inhaler *(continued)*

ACTION	**RATIONALE**
21. **Instruct patient to breathe in strong, steady and deeply through the mouth, for longer than 2 to 3 seconds.**	Activates the flow of medication. Deep inhalation allows for maximal distribution of medication to lung tissue.
22. Remove inhaler from mouth. Instruct patient to hold the breath for 5 to 10 seconds, or as long as possible, and then to exhale slowly through pursed lips.	This allows better distribution and longer absorption time for the medication.
23. Wait 1 to 5 minutes, as prescribed, before administering the next puff.	This ensures that both puffs are absorbed as much as possible. Bronchodilation after the first puff allows for deeper penetration by subsequent puffs.
24. After the prescribed number of puffs has been administered, have the patient replace the cap or storage container.	By replacing the cap, the patient is preventing any dust or dirt from entering the inhaler and being propelled into the bronchioles with later doses or from clogging the inhaler.
25. Have the patient gargle and rinse with tap water after using DPI, as necessary. Clean the DPI according to the manufacturer's directions.	Rinsing is necessary when using inhaled steroids, because oral fungal infections can occur. Rinsing removes medication residue from the mouth. Medication buildup in the device can affect how the medication is delivered, as well as attract bacteria.
26. Remove gloves and additional PPE, if used. Perform hand hygiene.	Proper removal of PPE reduces the risk for infection transmission and contamination of other items. Hand hygiene prevents the spread of microorganisms.
27. Document the administration of the medication immediately after administration. See Documentation section below.	Timely documentation helps to ensure patient safety.
28. Evaluate patient's response to the medication within an appropriate time frame. Reassess lung sounds, oxygen saturation level, and respirations, as indicated.	The patient needs to be evaluated for therapeutic and adverse effects from the medication. Lung sounds and oxygen saturation level may improve after DPI use. Respirations may decrease after DPI use.

EVALUATION

The expected outcomes have been achieved when the medication has been administered and breathed in by the patient; the patient experiences the intended effect of the medication; the patient understands the rationale for the inhaled medication; and the patient demonstrated correct use of the DPI.

DOCUMENTATION

Guidelines

Document the administration of the medication immediately after administration, including date, time, dose, and route of administration on the eMAR/MAR or record using the required format. If using a bar-code system, medication administration is automatically recorded when the bar code is scanned. PRN medications require documentation of the reason for administration. Prompt recording avoids the possibility of accidentally repeating the administration of the drug. Document respiratory rate, oxygen saturation, if applicable, lung assessment, and the patient's response to the treatment, if appropriate. If the drug was refused or omitted, record this in the appropriate area on the medication record and notify the primary care provider. This verifies the reason medication was omitted and ensures that health care personnel providing care for the patient are aware of the occurrence.

Sample Documentation

> 12/22/20 1715 Breath sounds slightly decreased in bases of lung pretreatment, respirations 18 breaths per minute and regular. After DPI, lung sounds remain diminished bilaterally in bases, O_2 saturation 97%, respiratory rate 16 breaths per minute. Patient able to demonstrate accurately the use of a DPI and verbalizes understanding of medication purpose and action.
>
> —C. Bausler, RN

UNEXPECTED SITUATIONS AND ASSOCIATED INTERVENTIONS

- *Patient reports that relief of symptoms has decreased:* Have patient demonstrate technique that he or she is using. Many patients develop poor habits over time (O'Conor et al., 2015). Poor administration technique can lead to a decrease in effectiveness of medication.

SPECIAL CONSIDERATIONS

General Considerations

- Instruct the patient never to exhale into the mouthpiece or shake the inhaler.
- If mist can be seen from the mouth or nose, the DPI is being used incorrectly.
- Follow the manufacturer's directions to clean the DPI.
- Store inhaler, capsules, and disks away from moisture at room temperature.
- Explain to the patient that there may not be any taste, smell, or feel associated with inhalation of the medication, which may be different from what they have experienced with another inhaler. As long as the directions for use of the DPI are followed, the patient will receive the full dose of medication (Cleveland Clinic, 2015).
- If the medication being administered is a steroid, the patient should rinse the mouth with water after administration to prevent irritation and secondary infection to the oral mucosa (Cleveland Clinic, 2015).
- Ongoing assessment is an important part of nursing care to evaluate patient response to administered medications and early detection of adverse drug reactions. If an adverse effect is suspected, withhold further medication doses and notify the patient's primary care provider. Additional intervention is based on type of reaction and patient assessment.

Home Care Considerations

- Many DPIs have dosage counters to keep track of remaining doses.
- If a particular DPI does not have a dose counter, teach patients how to tell when medication levels are getting low. The most reliable method is to look on the package and see how many doses the DPI contains. Divide this number by the number of doses used daily to ascertain how many days the DPI will last. Keep a diary or record of DPI use and discard the DPI on reaching the labeled number of doses.

EVIDENCE FOR PRACTICE ▶

INHALED MEDICATIONS

Correct use of a dry powder inhaler (DPI; diskus) is critical to ensure accurate dosing of medication. Patients who are prescribed medications delivered with a DPI must have accurate knowledge and demonstrate appropriate technique regarding use to ensure accurate medication delivery. Nurses play a key role in patient education and must have adequate knowledge to provide appropriate educational intervention.

Related Research

De Tratto, K., Gomez, C., Ryan, C. J., Bracken, N., Steffen, A., & Corbridge, S. J. (2014). Nurses' knowledge of inhaler technique in the inpatient hospital setting. *Clinical Nurse Specialist: The Journal for Advanced Nursing Practice, 28* (3), 156–160.

Refer to details in Skill 14, Evidence for Practice.

Skill 16 ▶ Administering Medication via a Small-Volume Nebulizer

Many medications prescribed for respiratory problems may be delivered via the respiratory system using a small-volume **nebulizer**. Nebulizers utilize the force of an oxygen stream or compressed air through a fluid medication to disperse fine particles of liquid medication into the deeper passages of the respiratory tract, where absorption occurs. The nebulizer medication treatment continues until all the medication in the nebulizer cup has been inhaled.

DELEGATION CONSIDERATIONS	The administration of medication via a nebulizer is not delegated to nursing assistive personnel (NAP) or to unlicensed assistive personnel (UAP). Depending on the state's nurse practice act and the organization's policies and procedures, administration of medication using a nebulizer may be delegated to licensed practical/vocational nurses (LPN/LVNs). The decision to delegate must be based on careful analysis of the patient's needs and circumstances, as well as the qualifications of the person to whom the task is being delegated.

EQUIPMENT

- Stethoscope
- Medication
- Nebulizer tubing and chamber
- Air compressor or oxygen hookup
- Sterile saline (if medication is not premeasured)
- Electronic Medication Administration Record (eMAR) or Medication Administration Record (MAR)
- PPE, as indicated

ASSESSMENT	Assess the appropriateness of the drug for the patient. Review medical history, allergy, assessment, and laboratory data that may influence drug administration. Assess respiratory rate, rhythm, and depth to establish a baseline. Assess lung sounds before and after use to establish a baseline and determine the effectiveness of the medication. Often, patients have wheezes or coarse lung sounds before medication administration. If ordered, assess patient's oxygen saturation level before medication administration. The oxygen saturation level may increase after the medication has been administered. Assess the patient's knowledge of the medication. If the patient has a knowledge deficit about the medication, this may be the appropriate time to begin education about the medication. If the medication may affect the patient's vital signs, assess them before administration. Verify patient name, dose, route, and time of administration.
NURSING DIAGNOSIS	Determine related factors for the nursing diagnoses based on the patient's current status. Appropriate nursing diagnoses may include: • Ineffective airway clearance • Impaired gas exchange • Ineffective breathing pattern
OUTCOME IDENTIFICATION AND PLANNING	The expected outcome to achieve is that the medication is administered and breathed in by the patient and the patient experiences the intended effect of the medication. Other outcomes that may be appropriate include the following: the patient understands the rationale for the inhaled medication; and the patient demonstrates correct use of the nebulizer.

IMPLEMENTATION

ACTION	RATIONALE
1. Gather equipment. Check each medication order against the original order in the health record, according to facility policy. Clarify any inconsistencies. Check the patient's health record for allergies.	This comparison helps to identify errors that may have occurred when orders were transcribed. The primary care provider's order or prescription/prescription is the legal record of medication orders for each facility.

ACTION	**RATIONALE**
2. Know the actions, special nursing considerations, safe dose ranges, purpose of administration, and adverse effects of the medications to be administered. Consider the appropriateness of the medication for this patient.	This knowledge aids the nurse in evaluating the therapeutic effect of the medication in relation to the patient's disorder and can also be used to educate the patient about the medication.
3. Perform hand hygiene.	Hand hygiene prevents the spread of microorganisms.
4. Move the medication supply system to the outside of the patient's room or prepare for administration at the medication supply system in the medication area. Alternatively, access the medication administration supply system at or inside the patient's room.	Organization facilitates error-free administration and saves time.
5. Unlock the medication supply system or drawer. Enter pass code and scan employee identification, if required.	Locking the medication supply system or drawer safeguards each patient's medication supply. Facility accrediting organizations require medication supply systems to be locked when not in use. Entering pass code and scanning ID allows only authorized users into the system and identifies the user for documentation by the computer.
6. **Prepare medications for one patient at a time.**	This prevents errors in medication administration.
7. Read the eMAR/MAR and select the proper medication from medication supply system or the patient's medication drawer.	This is the *first* check of the label.
8. Compare the label with the eMAR/MAR. Check expiration dates and perform calculations, if necessary. Scan the bar code on the package, if required.	This is the *second* check of the label. Verify calculations with another nurse to ensure safety, if necessary.
9. **Depending on facility policy, the third check of the label may occur at this point. If so, when all medications for one patient have been prepared, recheck the labels with the eMAR/MAR before taking the medications to the patient. However, many facilities require the third check to occur at the bedside, after identifying the patient.**	This *third* check ensures accuracy and helps to prevent errors. *Note:* Many facilities require the *third* check to occur at the bedside, after identifying the patient and before administration.
10. **Lock the medication supply system before leaving it.**	Locking the medication supply system or drawer safeguards the patient's medication supply. Facility accrediting organizations require medication supply systems to be locked when not in use.
11. Transport medications to the patient's bedside carefully, and keep the medications in sight at all times.	Careful handling and close observation prevent accidental or deliberate disarrangement of medications.
12. **Ensure that the patient receives the medications at the correct time.**	Check facility policy, which may allow for administration within a period of 30 minutes before or 30 minutes after the designated time.
13. Perform hand hygiene and put on PPE, if indicated.	Hand hygiene and PPE prevent the spread of microorganisms. PPE is required based on transmission precautions.

(continued)

Skill 16 ▶ Administering Medication via a Small-Volume Nebulizer *(continued)*

ACTION	RATIONALE

14. **Identify the patient. Compare the information with the eMAR/MAR. The patient should be identified using at least two of the following methods (The Joint Commission, 2018):**

Identifying the patient ensures the right patient receives the medications and helps prevent errors. The patient's room number or physical location is not used as an identifier (The Joint Commission, 2018). Replace the identification band if it is missing or inaccurate in any way.

a. Check the name on the patient's identification band.

b. Check the identification number on the patient's identification band.

c. Check the birth date on the patient's identification band.

d. Ask the patient to state his or her name and birth date, based on facility policy.

This requires a response from the patient, but illness and strange surroundings often cause patients to be confused.

15. **Complete necessary assessments before administering medications. Check the patient's allergy bracelet or ask the patient about allergies. Explain what you are going to do, and the reason for doing it, to the patient.**

Assessment is a prerequisite to administration of medications. Explanation relieves anxiety and facilitates cooperation.

16. Scan the patient's bar code on the identification band, if required.

Scanning provides an additional check to ensure that the medication is given to the right patient.

17. **Based on facility policy, the third check of the label may occur at this point. If so, recheck the labels with the eMAR/MAR before administering the medications to the patient.**

Many facilities require the *third* check to occur at the bedside, after identifying the patient and before administration. If facility policy directs the *third* check at this time, this *third* check ensures accuracy and helps to prevent errors.

18. Remove the nebulizer cup from the device and open it. Place premeasured unit-dose medication in the bottom section of the cup or use a dropper to place a concentrated dose of medication in the cup (Figure 1). Add prescribed diluent (usually saline), if required.

To get enough volume to make a fine mist, normal saline may need to be added to the concentrated medication.

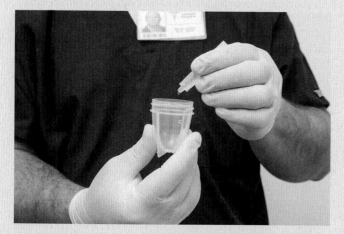

FIGURE 1. Putting medication into nebulizer.

19. Screw the top portion of the nebulizer cup back in place and attach the cup to the nebulizer. Attach one end of tubing to the stem on the bottom of the nebulizer cuff and the other end to the air compressor or oxygen source.

Air or oxygen must be forced through the nebulizer to form a fine mist.

20. Turn on the air compressor or oxygen. Check that a fine medication mist is produced by opening the valve. Have the patient place the mouthpiece into the mouth and grasp securely with teeth and lips.

If there is no fine mist, make sure that medication has been added to the cup and that the tubing is connected to the air compressor or oxygen outlet. Adjust flow meter if necessary.

ACTION	RATIONALE

21. Instruct the patient to inhale slowly and deeply through the mouth (Figure 2). A nose clip may be necessary if the patient is also breathing through the nose. Hold each breath for a slight pause, before exhaling.

While the patient inhales and holds the breath, the medication comes in contact with the respiratory tissue and is absorbed. The longer the breath is held, the more medication can be absorbed.

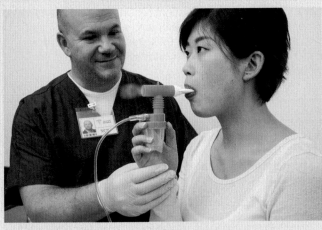

FIGURE 2. Inhaling slowly and deeply through the mouth.

22. Continue this inhalation technique until all medication in the nebulizer cup has been aerosolized (usually about 15 minutes). Once the fine mist decreases in amount, gently flick the sides of the nebulizer cup.

Once the fine mist stops, the medication is no longer being aerosolized. By gently flicking the cup sides, any medication that is stuck to the sides is knocked into the bottom of the cup, where it can become aerosolized.

23. When the medication in the nebulizer cup has been completely aerosolized, the cup will be empty. Have the patient remove the nebulizer from the mouth and gargle and rinse with tap water, as indicated. Clean and store the nebulizer and equipment according to the manufacturer's directions and facility policy.

Rinsing is necessary when using inhaled steroids, because oral fungal infections can occur. Rinsing removes medication residue from the mouth. The buildup of medication in the device can affect how the medication is delivered, as well as attract bacteria.

24. Remove gloves and additional PPE, if used. Perform hand hygiene.

Proper removal of PPE reduces the risk for infection transmission and contamination of other items. Hand hygiene prevents the spread of microorganisms.

25. Document the administration of the medication immediately after administration. See Documentation section below.

Timely documentation helps to ensure patient safety.

26. Evaluate patient's response to the medication within an appropriate time frame. Reassess lung sounds, oxygen saturation level, and respirations, as indicated.

The patient needs to be evaluated for therapeutic and adverse effects from the medication. Lung sounds and oxygen saturation level may improve after nebulizer use. Respirations may decrease after nebulizer use.

EVALUATION

The expected outcomes have been met when the medication has been administered and breathed in by the patient; the patient experiences the intended effect of the medication; the patient understands the rationale for the inhaled medication; and the patient demonstrated correct use of the nebulizer.

DOCUMENTATION

Guidelines

Document the administration of the medication immediately after administration, including date, time, dose, and route of administration on the eMAR/MAR or record using the required format. If using a bar-code system, medication administration is automatically recorded when the bar code is scanned. PRN medications require documentation of the reason for administration. Prompt recording avoids the possibility of accidentally repeating the administration of the drug. Document respiratory

(continued)

Skill 16 ▸ Administering Medication via a Small-Volume Nebulizer *(continued)*

rate, oxygen saturation, if applicable, lung assessment, and the patient's response to the treatment, if appropriate. If the drug was refused or omitted, record this in the appropriate area on the medication record and notify the primary care provider. This verifies the reason medication was omitted and ensures that health care personnel providing care for the patient are aware of the occurrence.

Sample Documentation

> <u>9/29/20</u> 2300 Wheezes noted in all lobes of lungs before albuterol nebulizer, O_2 saturation 92%, respiratory rate 24 breaths per minute, patient reports "feeling like I can't get my breath." Patient reassessed 20 minutes after albuterol nebulizer treatment; lung sounds are clear and equal in all lobes, O_2 saturation 97%, respiratory rate 18 breaths per minute unlabored. Patient verbalizes relief of shortness of breath and an understanding of medication purpose and action.
>
> —*C. Bausler, RN*

UNEXPECTED SITUATIONS AND ASSOCIATED INTERVENTIONS

- *Patient is unable to hold nebulizer in mouth and/or is unable to keep lips closed around device:* A plain oxygen mask can be attached to the nebulizer device and used to deliver the nebulized medication, eliminating the need to hold the device in the mouth.

SPECIAL CONSIDERATIONS

General Considerations

- Ongoing assessment is an important part of nursing care to evaluate patient response to administered medications and early detection of adverse drug reactions. If an adverse effect is suspected, withhold further medication doses and notify the patient's primary care provider. Additional intervention is based on type of reaction and patient assessment.

Infant and Child Considerations

- A small child may use a mask instead of a mouthpiece. Mask must fit securely over both the nose and the mouth to ensure a good seal and prevent medication escaping.
- Children must be able to seal their lips around the mouthpiece to use a nebulizer without a mask.

Home Care Considerations

- Medicine cup and mouthpiece should be washed with water and air dried (MedlinePlus, 2016d).

Skill 17 ▸ Administering Eye Drops

Eye drops are instilled for their local effects, such as for pupil dilation or constriction when examining the eye, for infection treatment, or for controlling intraocular pressure (e.g., for patients with glaucoma). The type and amount of solution administered depends on the purpose of the instillation.

The eye is a delicate organ, highly susceptible to infection and injury. Although the eye is never free of microorganisms, the secretions of the conjunctiva protect against many pathogens. For maximal safety for the patient, the equipment, solutions, and ointments introduced into the conjunctival sac should be sterile. If this is not possible, follow careful guidelines for medical asepsis. Refer to the accompanying Skill Variation for the steps to administer eye ointment.

DELEGATION CONSIDERATIONS

The administration of medication via drops in the eye is not delegated to nursing assistive personnel (NAP) or to unlicensed assistive personnel (UAP). Depending on the state's nurse practice act and the organization's policies and procedures, the administration of eye drops may be delegated to licensed practical/vocational nurses (LPN/LVNs). The decision to delegate must be based on careful analysis of the patient's needs and circumstances, as well as the qualifications of the person to whom the task is being delegated.

EQUIPMENT

- Gloves
- Additional PPE, as indicated
- Eye drop medication
- Tissues
- Normal saline solution

- Disposable washcloth, washcloth, cotton balls, or gauze squares
- Electronic Medication Administration Record (eMAR) or Medication Administration Record (MAR)

ASSESSMENT

Assess the appropriateness of the drug for the patient. Review medical history, allergy, assessment, and laboratory data that may influence drug administration. Check the expiration date before administering the medication. Assess the affected eye for any drainage, erythema, or swelling. Assess the patient's knowledge of the medication. If the patient has a knowledge deficit about the medication, this may be the appropriate time to begin education about the medication. Verify patient name, dose, route, and time of administration.

NURSING DIAGNOSIS

Determine related factors for the nursing diagnoses based on the patient's current status. Appropriate nursing diagnoses may include:

- Risk for allergy response
- Deficient knowledge
- Risk for injury

OUTCOME IDENTIFICATION AND PLANNING

The expected outcome to achieve when administering eye drops is that the medication is delivered successfully into the eye and the patient experiences the intended effect of the medication. Other outcomes that may be appropriate include the following: the patient experiences no allergy response; the patient does not exhibit systemic effects of the medication; the patient's eye remains free from injury; and patient understands the rationale for medication administration.

IMPLEMENTATION

ACTION	RATIONALE
1. Gather equipment. Check medication order against the original order in the health record, according to facility policy. Clarify any inconsistencies. Check the patient's health record for allergies.	This comparison helps to identify errors that may have occurred when orders were transcribed. The primary care provider's order or prescription is the legal record of medication orders for each facility.
2. Know the actions, special nursing considerations, safe dose ranges, purpose of administration, and adverse effects of the medications to be administered. Consider the appropriateness of the medication for this patient.	This knowledge aids the nurse in evaluating the therapeutic effect of the medication in relation to the patient's disorder and can also be used to educate the patient about the medication.
3. Perform hand hygiene.	Hand hygiene prevents the spread of microorganisms.
4. Move the medication supply system to the outside of the patient's room or prepare for administration at the medication supply system in the medication area. Alternatively, access the medication administration supply system at or inside the patient's room.	Organization facilitates error-free administration and saves time.
5. Unlock the medication supply system or drawer. Enter pass code and scan employee identification, if required.	Locking the medication supply system or drawer safeguards each patient's medication supply. Facility accrediting organizations require medication supply systems to be locked when not in use. Entering pass code and scanning ID allows only authorized users into the system and identifies the user for documentation by the computer.

(*continued*)

Skill 17 ▶ Administering Eye Drops *(continued)*

ACTION	**RATIONALE**
6. Prepare medications for one patient at a time.	This prevents errors in medication administration.
7. Read the eMAR/MAR and select the proper medication from the patient's medication drawer or medication supply system.	This is the *first* check of the label.
8. Compare the label with the eMAR/MAR. Check expiration dates and perform calculations, if necessary. Scan the bar code on the package, if required.	This is the *second* check of the label. Verify calculations with another nurse to ensure safety, if necessary.
9. Depending on facility policy, the third check of the label may occur at this point. If so, when all medications for one patient have been prepared, recheck the labels with the eMAR/MAR before taking the medications to the patient. However, many facilities require the third check to occur at the bedside, after identifying the patient.	This *third* check ensures accuracy and helps to prevent errors. *Note:* Many facilities require the *third* check to occur at the bedside, after identifying the patient and before administration.
10. Lock the medication supply system before leaving it.	Locking the medication supply system or drawer safeguards the patient's medication supply. Facility accrediting organizations require medication supply systems to be locked when not in use.
11. Transport medications to the patient's bedside carefully, and keep the medications in sight at all times.	Careful handling and close observation prevent accidental or deliberate disarrangement of medications.
12. Ensure that the patient receives the medications at the correct time.	Check facility policy, which may allow for administration within a period of 30 minutes before or 30 minutes after the designated time.
13. Perform hand hygiene and put on PPE, if indicated.	Hand hygiene and PPE prevent the spread of microorganisms. PPE is required based on transmission precautions.
14. Identify the patient. Compare the information with the eMAR/MAR. The patient should be identified using at least two of the following methods (The Joint Commission, 2018):	Identifying the patient ensures the right patient receives the medications and helps prevent errors. The patient's room number or physical location is not used as an identifier (The Joint Commission, 2018). Replace the identification band if it is missing or inaccurate in any way.
a. Check the name on the patient's identification band.	This requires a response from the patient, but illness and strange surroundings often cause patients to be confused.
b. Check the identification number on the patient's identification band.	
c. Check the birth date on the patient's identification band.	
d. Ask the patient to state his or her name and birth date, based on facility policy.	
15. Complete necessary assessments before administering medications. Check the patient's allergy bracelet or ask the patient about allergies. Explain the purpose and action of each medication to the patient.	Assessment is a prerequisite to administration of medications.
16. Scan the patient's bar code on the identification band, if required (Figure 1).	Provides an additional check to ensure that the medication is given to the right patient.
17. Based on facility policy, the third check of the label may occur at this point. If so, recheck the labels with the eMAR/MAR before administering the medications to the patient.	Many facilities require the *third* check to occur at the bedside, after identifying the patient and before administration. If facility policy directs the *third* check at this time, this *third* check ensures accuracy and helps to prevent errors.
18. Put on gloves.	Gloves protect the nurse from potential contact with mucous membranes and body fluids.
19. Offer tissue to patient.	Solution and tears may spill from the eye during the procedure.

ACTION

20. Cleanse the eyelids and eyelashes of any drainage with a washcloth, cotton balls, or gauze squares moistened with water or normal saline solution, as indicated by the patient's condition. Use each area of the cleaning surface once, moving from the inner toward the outer canthus (Figure 2).

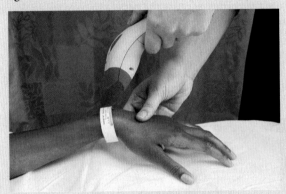

FIGURE 1. Scanning bar code on patient's identification bracelet.

21. Tilt the patient's head back slightly if sitting, or place the patient's head over a pillow if lying down. **Tilting the patient's head should be avoided if the patient has a cervical spine injury or other condition resulting in limited range-of-notion.** The head may be turned slightly to the affected side to prevent solution or tears from flowing toward the opposite eye (Figure 3).

22. Remove the cap from the medication bottle, being careful not to touch the inner side of the cap or the tip of the container. (See the accompanying Skill Variation for administering ointment.)

23. Invert the monodrip plastic container that is commonly used to instill eye drops. Have the patient look up and focus on something on the ceiling.

24. Place thumb or two fingers near margin of lower eyelid immediately below eyelashes, and apply pressure downward over bony cheek prominence. The lower conjunctival sac is exposed as the lower lid is pulled down (Figure 4).

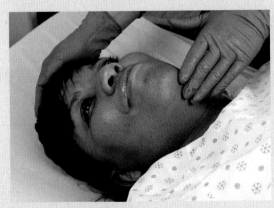

FIGURE 3. Turning head slightly to affected side.

RATIONALE

Debris can be carried into the eye when the conjunctival sac is exposed. Using each area of the gauze once and moving from the inner canthus to the outer canthus prevents carrying debris to the lacrimal ducts.

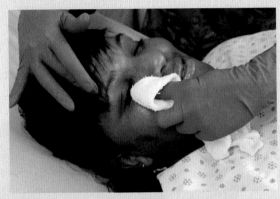

FIGURE 2. Cleaning eyelids and eyelashes from the inner toward the outer canthus.

Tilting the patient's head back slightly makes it easier to reach the conjunctival sac. Turning the head to the affected side helps to prevent solution or tears from flowing toward the opposite eye.

Touching the inner side of the cap or tip of container may contaminate the bottle of medication.

By having the patient look up and focus on something else, the procedure is less traumatic and keeps the eye still.

The eye drop should be placed in the conjunctival sac, not directly on the eyeball.

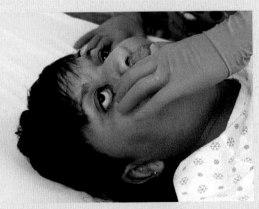

FIGURE 4. Applying pressure downward to expose lower conjunctival sac.

(continued)

Skill 17 ▶ Administering Eye Drops *(continued)*

ACTION	RATIONALE
25. Rest the lateral side of your hand on the patient's forehead, just above the eyebrow. **Hold the dropper close to the eye, but avoid touching eyelids or lashes.** Squeeze container and allow prescribed number of drops to fall in lower conjunctival sac (Figure 5).	Stabilizing hand on forehead prevents accidental contamination of the bottle tip and injury to the eye. Touching the eye, eyelids, or lashes can contaminate the medication in the bottle; startle the patient, causing blinking; or injure the eye. Do not allow medication to fall onto the cornea. This may injure the cornea or cause the patient to have an unpleasant sensation.
26. Release lower lid after eye drops are instilled. Ask patient to close eyes gently.	This allows the medication to be distributed over the entire eye.
27. Apply gentle pressure over inner canthus to prevent eye drops from flowing into tear duct (Figure 6).	This minimizes the risk of systemic effects from the medication.

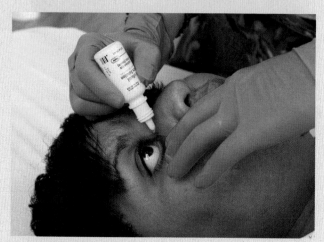

FIGURE 5. Squeezing container to administering drops into conjunctival sac.

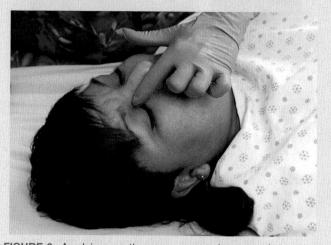

FIGURE 6. Applying gentle pressure over inner canthus.

28. Instruct patient not to rub affected eye. Replace the cover on the medication bottle.	This prevents injury and irritation to the eye. Cover prevents contamination.
29. Remove gloves. Assist the patient to a comfortable position.	This ensures patient comfort.
30. Remove additional PPE, if used. Perform hand hygiene.	Proper removal of PPE reduces the risk for infection transmission and contamination of other items. Hand hygiene prevents the spread of microorganisms.
31. Document the administration of the medication immediately after administration. See Documentation section below.	Timely documentation helps to ensure patient safety.
32. Evaluate the patient's response to the medication within an appropriate time frame.	The patient needs to be evaluated for therapeutic and adverse effects from the medication.

EVALUATION   The expected outcomes have been met when the medication is delivered successfully into the eye; the patient experiences the intended effect of the medication; the patient experiences no allergy response; the patient does not exhibit systemic effects of the medication; the patient's eye remains free from injury; and patient understands the rationale for medication administration.

DOCUMENTATION

Guidelines

Document the administration of the medication immediately after administration, including date, time, dose, route of administration, and site of administration, specifically right, left, or both eyes, on the eMAR/MAR or record using the required format. If using a bar-code system, medication administration is automatically recorded when the bar code is scanned. PRN medications require documentation of the reason for administration. Prompt recording avoids the possibility of accidentally repeating the administration of the drug. If the drug was refused or omitted, record this in the appropriate area on the medication record and notify the primary care provider. This verifies the reason medication was omitted and ensures that that health care personnel providing care for the patient are aware of the occurrence.

UNEXPECTED SITUATIONS AND ASSOCIATED INTERVENTIONS

- *Drop is placed on eyelid or outer margin of eyelid due to patient blinking or moving:* Do not count this drop in total number of drops administered. Allow the patient to regain composure and proceed with application of medication. Consider approaching the patient from below the line of sight.
- *You cannot open eyelids due to dried crust and matting of eyelids:* Place a warm, wet washcloth over the eye and allow it to remain there for approximately 3 minutes. Cleanse eye as described previously. You may need to repeat this procedure if there is a large amount of matting.
- *Bottle or tube of medication comes in contact with the eyeball when applying medication:* Bottle is contaminated; discard appropriately. Notify pharmacy or retrieve a new bottle.

SPECIAL CONSIDERATIONS

General Considerations

- Ongoing assessment is an important part of nursing care to evaluate patient response to administered medications and early detection of adverse drug reactions. If an adverse effect is suspected, withhold further medication doses and notify the patient's primary care provider. Additional intervention is based on type of reaction and patient assessment.

Infant and Child Considerations

- To apply eye drops in a small child, two or more people may be needed to restrain the child. Make sure the child does not reach up to the eye, causing the nurse to jab the medication bottle into the eye.

Skill Variation ▶ Administering Eye Ointment

Prepare medication as outlined in steps 1–21 above (Skill 17).

1. Have the patient look up and focus on something on the ceiling.
2. Place thumb or two fingers near margin of lower eyelid immediately below eyelashes and exert pressure downward over bony cheek prominence. Lower conjunctival sac is exposed as lower lid is pulled down.
3. Hold the ointment tube close to eye, but avoid touching eyelids or lashes. Squeeze container and apply about 0.5 in of ointment from the tube along the exposed sac. Apply the medication, moving from the inner canthus to the outer canthus. Twist tube to break off ribbon of ointment. **Do not touch the tip to the eye.**
4. Release lower lid after ointment is instilled. Ask the patient to close eyes gently.

5. The patient's body warmth helps to liquefy the ointment. Instruct the patient to keep the eye closed and move the eye in the socket to help to spread the ointment under the lids and over the surface of the eyeball. The patient may then open eye.
6. Assist the patient to a comfortable position. Explain that the ointment may temporarily blur vision; encourage the patient not to rub the eye.
7. Remove gloves and additional PPE, if used. Perform hand hygiene.
8. Document administration of the medication on the eMAR/MAR immediately after administering the medication.
9. Evaluate the patient's response to the medication within an appropriate time frame.

Skill 18 ▶ Administering Ear Drops

Drugs are instilled into the auditory canal for their local effect. They are used to soften wax, relieve pain, apply local anesthesia, and treat infections. If the tympanic membrane is ruptured or has been opened by surgical intervention, the middle ear and the inner ear have a direct passage to the external ear. When this occurs, perform instillations with the greatest of care to prevent forcing materials from the outer ear into the middle ear and the inner ear. Use sterile technique to prevent infection.

DELEGATION CONSIDERATIONS

The administration of medication via drops in the ear is not delegated to nursing assistive personnel (NAP) or to unlicensed assistive personnel (UAP). Depending on the state's nurse practice act and the organization's policies and procedures, the administration of ear drop may be delegated to licensed practical/vocational nurses (LPN/LVNs). The decision to delegate must be based on careful analysis of the patient's needs and circumstances, as well as the qualifications of the person to whom the task is being delegated.

EQUIPMENT

- Ear drop medication (warmed to 98.6°F [37°C])
- Tissue
- Cotton balls (optional)
- Gloves
- Additional PPE, as indicated
- Disposable washcloth or washcloth (optional)
- Normal saline solution or warm water
- Electronic Medication Administration Record (eMAR) or Medication Administration Record (MAR)

ASSESSMENT

Assess the appropriateness of the drug for the patient. Review medical history, allergy, assessment, and laboratory data that may influence drug administration. Assess the affected ear for redness, erythema, edema, drainage, or tenderness. Assess the patient's knowledge of medication and procedure. If the patient has a knowledge deficit about the medication, this may be an appropriate time to begin education about the medication. Assess the patient's ability to cooperate with the procedure. Verify patient name, dose, route, and time of administration.

NURSING DIAGNOSIS

Determine related factors for the nursing diagnoses based on the patient's current status. Appropriate nursing diagnoses may include:

- Deficient knowledge
- Risk for injury
- Acute pain

OUTCOME IDENTIFICATION AND PLANNING

The expected outcome to achieve is that drops are administered successfully and the patient experiences the intended effect of the medication. Other outcomes that may be appropriate include the following: the patient understands the rationale for the ear drop instillation; and the patient does not experience injury.

IMPLEMENTATION

ACTION	RATIONALE
1. Gather equipment. Check medication order against the original order in the health record, according to facility policy. Clarify any inconsistencies. Check the patient's health record for allergies.	This comparison helps to identify errors that may have occurred when orders were transcribed. The primary care provider's order or prescription is the legal record of medication orders for each facility.
2. Know the actions, special nursing considerations, safe dose ranges, purpose of administration, and adverse effects of the medication to be administered. Consider the appropriateness of the medication for this patient.	This knowledge aids the nurse in evaluating the therapeutic effect of the medication in relation to the patient's disorder and can also be used to educate the patient about the medication.

ACTION	RATIONALE

3. Perform hand hygiene.

Hand hygiene prevents the spread of microorganisms.

4. Move the medication supply system to the outside of the patient's room or prepare for administration at the medication supply system in the medication area. Alternatively, access the medication administration supply system at or inside the patient's room.

Organization facilitates error-free administration and saves time.

5. Unlock the medication supply system or drawer. Enter pass code and scan employee identification, if required.

Locking the medication supply system or drawer safeguards each patient's medication supply. Facility accrediting organizations require medication supply systems to be locked when not in use. Entering pass code and scanning ID allows only authorized users into the system and identifies the user for documentation by the computer.

6. **Prepare medications for one patient at a time.**

This prevents errors in medication administration.

7. Read the eMAR/MAR and select the proper medication from the patient's medication drawer or medication supply system.

This is the *first* check of the label.

8. Compare the label with the eMAR/MAR. Check expiration dates and perform calculations, if necessary. Scan the bar code on the package, if required.

This is the *second* check of the label. Verify calculations with another nurse to ensure safety, if necessary.

9. **Depending on facility policy, the third check of the label may occur at this point. If so, when all medications for one patient have been prepared, recheck the labels with the eMAR/MAR before taking the medications to the patient. However, many facilities require the third check to occur at the bedside, after identifying the patient.**

This *third* check ensures accuracy and helps to prevent errors. *Note:* Many facilities require the *third* check to occur at the bedside, after identifying the patient and before administration.

10. **Lock the medication supply system before leaving it.**

Locking the medication supply system or drawer safeguards the patient's medication supply. Facility accrediting organizations require medication supply systems to be locked when not in use.

11. Transport medications to the patient's bedside carefully, and keep the medications in sight at all times.

Careful handling and close observation prevent accidental or deliberate disarrangement of medications.

12. **Ensure that the patient receives the medications at the correct time.**

Check facility policy, which may allow for administration within a period of 30 minutes before or 30 minutes after the designated time.

13. Perform hand hygiene and put on PPE, if indicated.

Hand hygiene and PPE prevent the spread of microorganisms. PPE is required based on transmission precautions.

14. **Identify the patient. Compare the information with the eMAR/MAR. The patient should be identified using at least two of the following methods (The Joint Commission, 2018):**

Identifying the patient ensures the right patient receives the medications and helps prevent errors. The patient's room number or physical location is not used as an identifier (The Joint Commission, 2018). Replace the identification band if it is missing or inaccurate in any way.

a. Check the name on the patient's identification band.

b. Check the identification number on the patient's identification band.

c. Check the birth date on the patient's identification band.

d. Ask the patient to state his or her name and birth date, based on facility policy.

This requires a response from the patient, but illness and strange surroundings often cause patients to be confused.

(continued)

Skill 18 ▶ Administering Ear Drops *(continued)*

ACTION	RATIONALE
15. Complete necessary assessments before administering medications. Check the patient's allergy bracelet or ask the patient about allergies. Explain the purpose and action of each medication to the patient.	Assessment is a prerequisite to administration of medications.
16. Scan the patient's bar code on the identification band, if required.	Provides an additional check to ensure that the medication is given to the right patient.
17. Based on facility policy, the third check of the label may occur at this point. If so, recheck the labels with the eMAR/MAR before administering the medications to the patient.	Many facilities require the *third* check to occur at the bedside, after identifying the patient and before administration. If facility policy directs the *third* check at this time, this *third* check ensures accuracy and helps to prevent errors.
18. Put on gloves.	Gloves protect the nurse from potential contact with mucous membranes and body fluids.
19. Cleanse external ear of any drainage with cotton ball or washcloth moistened with normal saline or water (Figure 1).	Debris and drainage may prevent some of the medication from entering the ear canal.
20. Place patient on his or her unaffected side in bed, or, if ambulatory, have patient sit with head well tilted to the side so that the affected ear is uppermost (Figure 2).	This positioning prevents the drops from escaping from the ear.

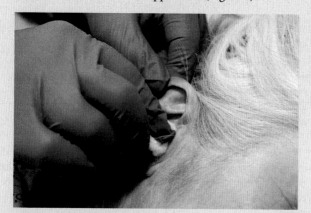

FIGURE 1. Cleaning external ear.

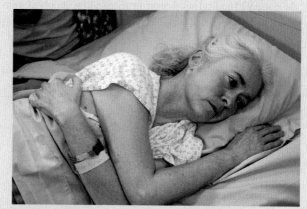

FIGURE 2. Positioning patient on unaffected side.

21. Remove the cap from the medication bottle, being careful not to touch the inner side of the cap or the tip of the container (Figure 3).	Touching the inner side of the cap or tip of container may contaminate the bottle of medication.

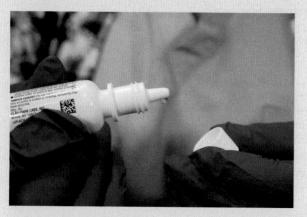

FIGURE 3. Removing the cap from the medication bottle.

22. Straighten auditory canal by pulling cartilaginous portion of pinna up and back for an adult. (See Infant and Child Considerations for correct positioning for this age group.)	Pulling on the pinna as described helps to straighten the canal properly for ear drop instillation.

ACTION	RATIONALE
23. Invert and hold medication bottle in the ear with its tip above the auditory canal (Figure 4). Do not touch the dropper to the ear.	By holding the medication bottle in the ear, the medication will enter the ear canal. Touching the bottle to the ear contaminates the bottle and medication. The hard tip of the medication bottle can damage the tympanic membrane if it is jabbed into the ear.

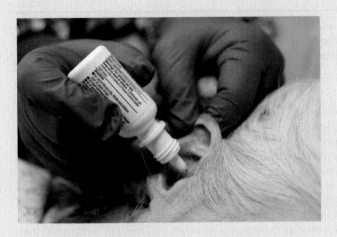

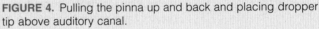
FIGURE 4. Pulling the pinna up and back and placing dropper tip above auditory canal.

24. **Squeeze container and allow drops to fall on the side of the canal. Avoid instilling in the middle of the canal, to avoid instilling directly onto the tympanic membrane.**	It is uncomfortable for the patient if the drops fall directly onto the tympanic membrane.
25. Release pinna after instilling drops, and have patient maintain the head position to prevent escape of medication.	Medication should remain in ear canal for at least 5 minutes.
26. Gently press on the tragus a few times (Figure 5).	Pressing on the tragus causes medication from the canal to move toward the tympanic membrane.
27. If ordered, loosely insert a cotton ball into the ear canal (Figure 6).	A cotton ball can help prevent medication from leaking out of the ear canal.

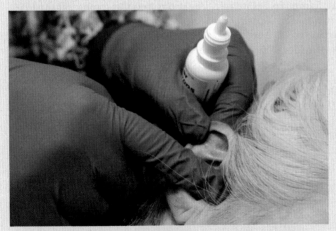
FIGURE 5. Applying pressure to tragus.

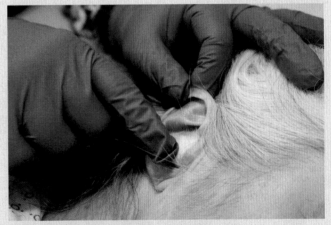
FIGURE 6. Inserting cotton ball into ear canal.

28. Instruct patient to remain lying down with the affected ear upward for 5 minutes.	This ensures medication remains in ear canal.
29. Replace cap on medication bottle. Remove gloves and additional PPE, if used. Perform hand hygiene.	Replacing cap prevents contamination of tip of bottle. Proper removal of PPE reduces the risk for infection transmission and contamination of other items. Hand hygiene prevents the spread of microorganisms.

(continued)

Skill 18 ▶ Administering Ear Drops *(continued)*

ACTION	RATIONALE
30. Document the administration of the medication immediately after administration. See Documentation section below.	Timely documentation helps to ensure patient safety.
31. Evaluate the patient's response to medication within an appropriate time frame.	The patient needs to be evaluated for therapeutic and adverse effects from the medication.

EVALUATION

The expected outcomes have been met when the ear drops have been administered successfully; the patient experiences the intended effect of the medication; the patient understands the rationale for the ear drop instillation; and the patient did not experience injury.

DOCUMENTATION

Guidelines

Document the administration of the medication immediately after administration, including date, time, dose, route of administration, and site of administration, specifically right, left, or both ears, on the eMAR/MAR or record using the required format. If using a bar-code system, medication administration is automatically recorded when the bar code is scanned. PRN medications require documentation of the reason for administration. Prompt recording avoids the possibility of accidentally repeating the administration of the drug. Document pre- and post-administration assessments, characteristics of any drainage, and the patient's response to the treatment, if appropriate. If the drug was refused or omitted, record this in the appropriate area on the medication record and notify the primary care provider. This verifies the reason medication was omitted and ensures that health care personnel providing care for the patient are aware of the occurrence.

UNEXPECTED SITUATIONS AND ASSOCIATED INTERVENTIONS

- *Medication runs from ear into eye:* Notify primary care provider and check with the pharmacy. Eye irrigation may need to be performed.
- *Patient complains of extreme pain when you press on the tragus:* Allow patient to press on tragus. If pressure causes too much pain, this part may be deferred.

SPECIAL CONSIDERATIONS

General Considerations

- If both ears are to be treated, wait 5 minutes before instilling drops into the second ear.
- Ongoing assessment is an important part of nursing care to evaluate patient response to administered treatments and early detection of adverse drug reactions. If an adverse effect is suspected, notify the patient's primary care provider. Additional intervention is based on type of reaction and patient assessment.

Infant and Child Considerations

- Pull pinna up and back for a child older than 3 years (Figure 7) and down and back for an infant or a child younger than 3 years (Figure 8) (Kee et al., 2015; Kyle & Carman, 2017).
- Distraction techniques, such as TV or a quiet toy, may be helpful when attempting to keep a child quiet for 5 minutes. Reading to the child may not be appropriate because the child's hearing may be compromised during medication administration.

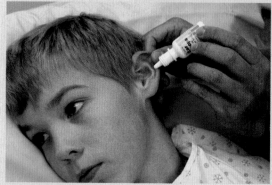

FIGURE 7. Pulling pinna up and back for a child older than 3 years.

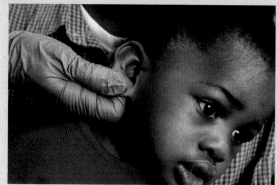

FIGURE 8. Pulling pinna down and back for an infant or child younger than 3 years.

Skill 19 ▶ Administering a Nasal Spray

Nasal instillations are used to treat allergies, sinus infections, and nasal congestion. Medications with a systemic effect, such as vasopressin, may also be prepared as a nasal instillation. The nose is normally not a sterile cavity, but because of its connection with the sinuses, it is important to observe medical asepsis carefully when using nasal instillations.

The following skill describes the steps to administer a nasal spray. Refer to the accompanying Skill Variation for guidelines to administer medication via nasal drops.

DELEGATION CONSIDERATIONS	The administration of medication using a nasal spray is not delegated to nursing assistive personnel (NAP) or to unlicensed assistive personnel (UAP). Depending on the state's nurse practice act and the organization's policies and procedures, administration of a nasal spray may be delegated to licensed practical/vocational nurses (LPN/LVNs). The decision to delegate must be based on careful analysis of the patient's needs and circumstances, as well as the qualifications of the person to whom the task is being delegated.
EQUIPMENT	• Medication in nasal spray bottle • Gloves • Additional PPE, as indicated • Tissue • Electronic Medication Administration Record (eMAR) or Medication Administration Record (MAR)
ASSESSMENT	Assess the appropriateness of the drug for the patient. Review medical history, allergy, assessment, and laboratory data that may influence drug administration. Assess the nares for redness, erythema, edema, drainage, or tenderness. Assess the patient's knowledge of medication and the procedure. If the patient has a knowledge deficit about the medication, this may be an appropriate time to begin education about the procedure. Assess the patient's ability to cooperate with the procedure. Verify patient name, dose, route, and time of administration.
NURSING DIAGNOSIS	Determine related factors for the nursing diagnoses based on the patient's current status. Appropriate nursing diagnoses may include: • Deficient knowledge •Risk for allergy reaction
OUTCOME IDENTIFICATION AND PLANNING	The expected outcome to achieve is that the medication is administered successfully into the nose and the patient experiences the intended effect of the medication. Other outcomes that may be appropriate include the following: the patient understands the rationale for the nose spray; the patient experiences no allergy response; and the patient experiences minimal discomfort.

IMPLEMENTATION

ACTION	RATIONALE
1. Gather equipment. Check medication order against the original order in the health record, according to facility policy. Clarify any inconsistencies. Check the patient's health record for allergies.	This comparison helps to identify errors that may have occurred when orders were transcribed. The primary care provider's order or prescription is the legal record of medication orders for each facility.
2. Know the actions, special nursing considerations, safe dose ranges, purpose of administration, and adverse effects of the medication to be administered. Consider the appropriateness of the medication for this patient.	This knowledge aids the nurse in evaluating the therapeutic effect of the medication in relation to the patient's disorder and can also be used to educate the patient about the medication.
3. Perform hand hygiene.	Hand hygiene prevents the spread of microorganisms.

(continued)

Skill 19 ▶ Administering a Nasal Spray *(continued)*

ACTION	**RATIONALE**
4. Move the medication supply system to the outside of the patient's room or prepare for administration at the medication supply system in the medication area. Alternatively, access the medication administration supply system at or inside the patient's room.	Organization facilitates error-free administration and saves time.
5. Unlock the medication supply system or drawer. Enter pass code and scan employee identification, if required.	Locking the medication supply system or drawer safeguards each patient's medication supply. Facility accrediting organizations require medication supply systems to be locked when not in use. Entering pass code and scanning ID allows only authorized users into the system and identifies the user for documentation by the computer.
6. Prepare medications for one patient at a time.	This prevents errors in medication administration.
7. Read the eMAR/MAR and select the proper medication from the patient's medication drawer or medication supply system.	This is the *first* check of the label.
8. Compare the label with the eMAR/MAR. Check expiration dates and perform calculations, if necessary. Scan the bar code on the package, if required.	This is the *second* check of the label. Verify calculations with another nurse to ensure safety, if necessary.
9. Depending on facility policy, the third check of the label may occur at this point. If so, when all medications for one patient have been prepared, recheck the labels with the eMAR/MAR before taking the medications to the patient. However, many facilities require the third check to occur at the bedside, after identifying the patient.	This *third* check ensures accuracy and helps to prevent errors. *Note:* Many facilities require the *third* check to occur at the bedside, after identifying the patient and before administration.
10. Lock the medication supply system before leaving it.	Locking the medication supply system or drawer safeguards the patient's medication supply. Facility accrediting organizations require medication supply systems to be locked when not in use.
11. Transport medications to the patient's bedside carefully, and keep the medications in sight at all times.	Careful handling and close observation prevent accidental or deliberate disarrangement of medications.
12. Ensure that the patient receives the medications at the correct time.	Check facility policy, which may allow for administration within a period of 30 minutes before or 30 minutes after the designated time.
13. Perform hand hygiene and put on PPE, if indicated.	Hand hygiene and PPE prevent the spread of microorganisms. PPE is required based on transmission precautions.
14. Identify the patient. Compare the information with the eMAR/MAR. The patient should be identified using at least two of the following methods (The Joint Commission, 2018):	Identifying the patient ensures the right patient receives the medications and helps prevent errors. The patient's room number or physical location is not used as an identifier (The Joint Commission, 2018). Replace the identification band if it is missing or inaccurate in any way.
a. Check the name on the patient's identification band. b. Check the identification number on the patient's identification band. c. Check the birth date on the patient's identification band. d. Ask the patient to state his or her name and birth date, based on facility policy.	This requires a response from the patient, but illness and strange surroundings often cause patients to be confused.
15. Complete necessary assessments before administering medications. Check the patient's allergy bracelet or ask the patient about allergies. Explain the purpose and action of each medication to the patient.	Assessment is a prerequisite to administration of medications.

ACTION

16. Scan the patient's bar code on the identification band, if required (Figure 1).

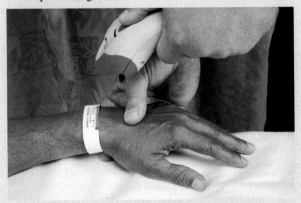

FIGURE 1. Scanning bar code on the patient's identification bracelet.

17. Based on facility policy, the third check of the label may occur at this point. If so, recheck the labels with the eMAR/MAR before administering the medications to the patient.

18. Put on gloves.

19. Provide patient with paper tissues and ask the patient to blow his or her nose.

20. Have the patient sit up with head tilted back. **Tilting the patient's head should be avoided if the patient has a cervical spine injury or other condition resulting in limited range of notion.**

21. Instruct the patient that it is necessary to inhale gently through the nose as the spray is being administered or not to inhale gently as the spray is being administered. Your instruction to the patient will depend on the medication being administered. Consult the manufacturer's instructions for each medication.

22. Agitate the bottle gently, if required for specific medication. Insert the tip of the nosepiece of the bottle into one nostril (Figure 2). Close the opposite nostril with a finger. Instruct the patient to breathe in gently through the nostril, if required. Compress or activate the bottle to release one spray at the same time the patient breathes in.

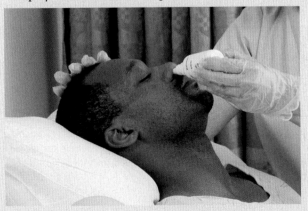

FIGURE 2. Inserting tip of bottle into one nostril.

RATIONALE

Provides an additional check to ensure that the medication is given to the right patient.

Many facilities require the *third* check to occur at the bedside, after identifying the patient and before administration. If facility policy directs the *third* check at this time, this *third* check ensures accuracy and helps to prevent errors.

Gloves protect the nurse from potential contact with contaminants and body fluids.

Blowing the nose clears the nasal mucosa prior to medication administration.

Allows the spray to flow into the nares. Tilting the head is contraindicated with cervical spine injury.

Inhalation helps to distribute the spray in the nares. Inhalation during administration is not recommended for some medications.

Mixes medication thoroughly to ensure a consistent dose of medication.

(continued)

Skill 19 ▶ Administering a Nasal Spray (continued)

ACTION	RATIONALE
23. Keep the medication container compressed and remove it from the nostril. Release the container from the compressed state. Do not allow the container to return to its original position until it is removed from the patient's nose.	Prevents contamination of the contents of the container.
24. Have the patient hold his or her breath for a few seconds, and then breathe out slowly through the mouth. Repeat in the other nostril, as prescribed or indicated.	Allows medication to remain in contact with mucous membranes of nose.
25. Wipe the outside of the bottle nose piece with a clean, dry tissue or cloth and replace the cap. Instruct the patient to avoid blowing his or her nose for 5 to 10 minutes, depending on the medication.	Keeps the end of the bottle clean. Keeps the medication in contact with the mucous membranes of the nose.
26. Remove gloves. Assist the patient to a comfortable position.	This ensures patient comfort.
27. Remove additional PPE, if used. Perform hand hygiene.	Proper removal of PPE reduces the risk for infection transmission and contamination of other items. Hand hygiene prevents the spread of microorganisms.
28. Document the administration of the medication immediately after administration. See Documentation section below.	Timely documentation helps to ensure patient safety.
29. Evaluate the patient's response to the procedure and medication within an appropriate time frame.	The patient needs to be evaluated for therapeutic and adverse effects from the medication.

EVALUATION

The expected outcomes have been met when the medication has been administered successfully into the nose; the patient experiences the intended effect of the medication; the patient understands the rationale for the nose spray; the patient experiences no allergy response; and the patient experienced minimal discomfort.

DOCUMENTATION

Guidelines

Document the administration of the medication, including date, time, dose, route of administration, and site of administration, specifically right, left, or both nares, on the eMAR/MAR or record using the required format. If using a bar-code system, medication administration is automatically recorded when the bar code is scanned. PRN medications require documentation of the reason for administration. Prompt recording avoids the possibility of accidentally repeating the administration of the drug. Document pre- and post-administration assessments, characteristics of any drainage, and the patient's response to the treatment, if appropriate. If the drug was refused or omitted, record this in the appropriate area on the medication record and notify the primary care provider. This verifies the reason medication was omitted and ensures that health care personnel providing care for the patient are aware of the occurrence.

UNEXPECTED SITUATIONS AND ASSOCIATED INTERVENTIONS

- *Patient sneezes immediately after receiving nose spray:* Do not repeat the dosage, because you cannot determine how much medication was actually absorbed.

SPECIAL CONSIDERATIONS

- Ongoing assessment is an important part of nursing care to evaluate patient response to administered medications and early detection of adverse drug reactions. If an adverse effect is suspected, withhold further medication doses and notify the patient's primary care provider. Additional intervention is based on type of reaction and patient assessment.

Skill Variation ▶ Administering Medication via Nasal Drops

Prepare medication as outlined in steps 1–17 above (Skill 19).

1. Put on gloves. Assist the patient to an upright position with the head tilted back.
2. Draw sufficient solution into the dropper for both nares. Do not return excess solution to the bottle to avoid contamination.
3. Have the patient breathe through the mouth. Hold tip of nose up and place dropper just above naris, about 1/3 in. Instill the prescribed number of drops in one naris and then into the other. Avoid touching naris with dropper.

4. Have patient remain in position with head tilted back for 5 minutes to prevent the escape of the medication.
5. Remove gloves and any additional PPE, if used. Perform hand hygiene.

6. Document administration of the medication on the eMAR/MAR immediately after administering the medication. Document the site, if only one nostril is used.
7. Evaluate the patient's response to the medication within an appropriate time frame.